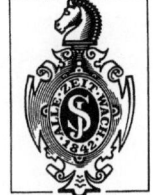

G. E. Fackelman   D. M. Nunamaker

Manual of Internal Fixation in the Horse

In Collaboration with B. von Salis and O. Pohler

Foreword by M. E. Müller, M. Allgöwer,
R. Schneider, H. Willenegger

With 187 Figures in 282 Separate Illustrations

Springer-Verlag
Berlin Heidelberg New York 1982

Gustave E. Fackelman, D.V.M.
Professor of Surgery
Tufts University
School of Veterinary Medicine
Westboro Road
North Grafton, MA 01536/USA

David M. Nunamaker, V.M.D.
Jacques Jenny Associate Professor
of Orthopaedic Surgery
School of Veterinary Medicine
New Bolton Center
Kennett Square, PA 19348/USA

Illustrations by E. J. Michener

ISBN-13:978-3-642-81471-6   e-ISBN-13:978-3-642-81469-3
DOI:10.1007/978-3-642-81469-3

Library of Congress Cataloging in Publication Data. Fackelman, Gustave E. 1941–. Manual
of internal fixation in the horse. Bibliography: p. Includes index. 1. Horses-Surgery. 2. Internal fixation in fractures. 3. Fractures in animals. I. Nunamaker, David M., 1944–. joint
author. II. Title. SF914.4.F32. 636.1′089715. 80-27316

2124/3140-543210

In Memory of
Prof. Jacques Jenny

Foreword

It is with pleasure that we offer these introductory remarks for the Manual of Internal Fixation in the Horse, a book describing a further application of AO or ASIF techniques. The letters A-O stand for the Arbeitsgemeinschaft für Osteosynthesefragen and have been translated into the Association for the Study of Internal Fixation. The organization is truly a "study group", created in Switzerland, that met for the first time in 1958. The major goal was to establish a task force committed to the improvement of fracture treatment by osteosynthesis.

The group's motivation arose out of the then prevailing unsound or inconsistently successful attempts at fracture treatment. According to statistics obtained from the Swiss National Health Insurance Program at the time, the so-called conservative treatment of fractures had resulted in a high rate of persistent morbidity. The problems encountered included: irreparable damage due to long-term immobilization; delayed union or pseudoarthrosis; malalignment; and, inadequate reduction of intraarticular fractures with resultant osteoarthritis. Accurate, stable osteosynthesis seemed the only practical way to address those various shortcomings. However, many of the osteosyntheses performed at that time had led to new problems, since most were not stable and, in some cases, actually worked to prevent healing. In those cases, external immobilization, with all its inherent drawbacks, again became necessary. This set of circumstances seemed particularly common when cerclage was used in the repair of long bone fractures. When inadequate technique was complicated by postoperative infection, the outcome was disastrous; and it is no surprise that there were many opponents to any plan designed to further the development of internal fixation.

Against this background the AO group set out to find, based on solid scientific evidence, a way to perform osteosynthesis with an absolute minimum of complications. Through close cooperation between surgeons, basic researchers, metallurgists, and statisticians, our goal was achieved and osteosynthesis has been standardized as a surgical method. The techniques developed were applicable not only to fracture treatment, but also to many other areas in the surgery of the locomotor system. Along with the basic principle of absolute stability in internal fixation, early postoperative mobilization and even weight-

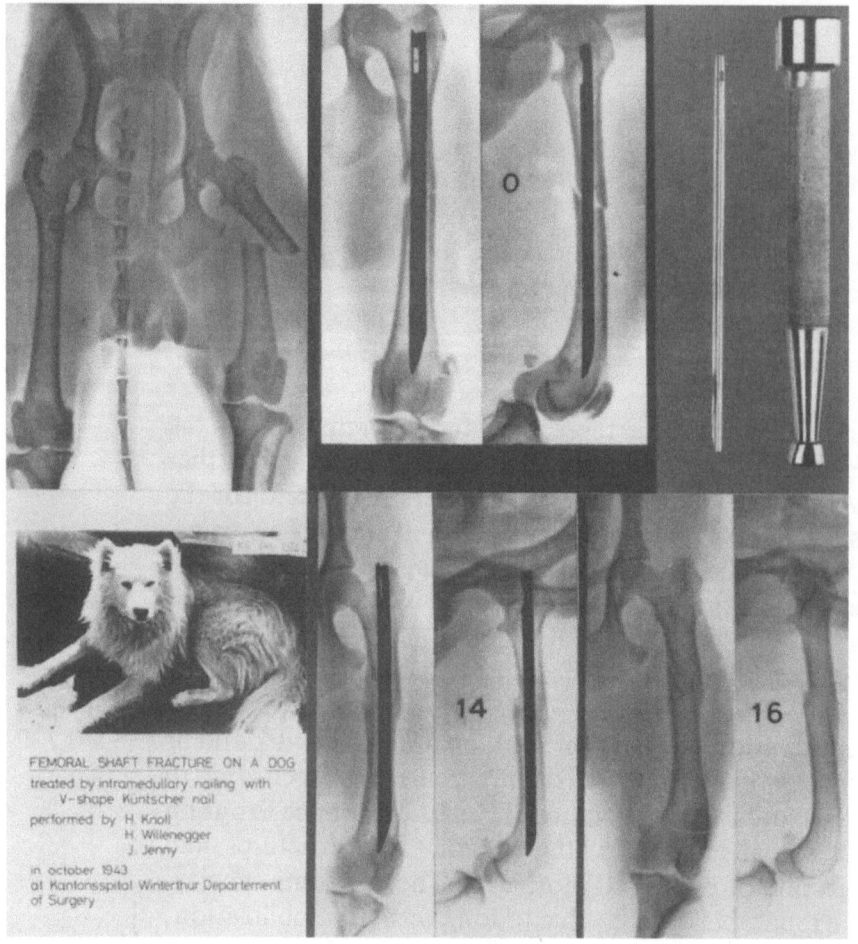

FEMORAL SHAFT FRACTURE ON A DOG
treated by intramedullary nailing with
V-shape Kuntscher nail

performed by H. Knoll
H. Willenegger
J. Jenny

in october 1943
at Kantonsspital Winterthur Departement
of Surgery

bearing played an important role in bringing about a positive outcome. This latter point seemed particularly important in stimulating the expansion of operative treatment of fractures into clinical veterinary surgery.

In Switzerland, intramedullary nailing found immediate acceptance, the first dog having been treated by the technique in October 1943. The case in question had historical implications, in that it was carried out with the help of Dr. Jacques Jenny, then a resident at the University of Zurich and a man that would later play a key role in the refinement of internal fixation, especially in large animals. The first plate fixation in animals in Switzerland was performed by Dr. R. Fischer, an AO member, in collaboration with a veterinarian, Dr. Eppenburger. The implants were applied to successfully repair fractures of the mandible in two oxen.

Eighteen years after the above-mentioned canine intramedullary nailing, further decisive contacts were established. Dr. Howard Rosen and Dr. Bruce Hohn first met at the Annual Congress of the American Academy of Orthopedic Surgeons in January 1965. Hohn was at that time the Head of the Surgical Section at the Animal Medical Center in

New York, where Rosen was soon thereafter appointed as consultant. Later that year Dr. Jacques Jenny became acquainted with the former two individuals and a nucleus was formed around which other colleagues soon gathered.

The founders of the AO owe a vote of thanks of their veterinary colleagues, who have helped immeasurably through clinical work and basic research to advance the high standards we now enjoy. The authors of the Manual der Osteosynthese wish the authors of this present volume every success and trust that the book will find enthusiastic acceptance and broad application.

M. E. Müller
M. Allgöwer
R. Schneider
H. Willenegger

Preface

In the 1960s, veterinarians became aware of a system of fracture treatment developed by the AO (Arbeitsgemeinschaft für Osteosynthesefragen), a Swiss group of surgeons dedicated to the improvement of internal fixation devices and techniques for the treatment of fractures in humans. The basic goals of the group, which rapidly developed an American counterpart, the ASIF (Association for the Study of Internal Fixation), seemed very similar to our own: early post-operative weight bearing; accurate reconstruction; healing with minimal callus; and the elimination of joint stiffness and "fracture disease."

It was therefore not surprising to see reports appearing in veterinary journals and conference proceedings of the use of ASIF techniques in animals by such pioneers as Jacques Jenny, Wade Brinker and R. Bruce Hohn. In 1967, these veterinarians and several others attended a short course designed to introduce the AO technique to physicians. The following year special courses for a small number of veterinarians were set up in Davos, Switzerland, and in Columbus, Ohio, and "AO Vet." groups began to form on both sides of the Atlantic.

Acknowledging the youth of the field and the present shortcomings of fracture treatment in the horse, it is our purpose to set out in print the principles of internal fixation, using case illustrations to describe the techniques which have been most successful. It is not the purpose of this book to exclude the techniques of others, nor to imply that techniques which have not been included are unsatisfactory, it is just that the ones presented here have been used by either one or both of us, and, since they are based on a certain degree of satisfactory results, are considered important enough to be included. Not all fractures are identical as they present themselves clinically, and subtle variations in form may require modifications or combinations of techniques to produce the desired end-result. *Stability* of the fracture fragments relative to one another is the keynote to healing. This is more important in horses than in other species, since the stresses to be withstood by the implants are much greater and the rate of healing of bone may be, according to some preliminary work, slower than in other animals studied.

When assessing the case material presented, it is noted that most of the techniques described are limited to screw fixation. This method, together with plate fixation, is frequently used in long-bone fractures in the horse. Shaft fractures are covered in the general discussion of Part I and are not covered bone by bone in the more specilized Part II. This has been done so that the principles of internal fixation can be followed even though there are such great variations between individual bones and degrees of injury. No detailed instructions are given for shaft fractures since success will depend on the skill and experience of each surgeon. Not all shaft fractures are presently amenable to treatment.

This manual serves to describe the implements and techniques of internal fixation in large animals to the best of our knowledge at the time of publication. Though the illustrations and text deal only with horses, most of the techniques and all of the principles apply equally to other large domestic and exotic animal species. The book will be especially useful to anyone who has participated in practical courses teaching the ASIF method. Readers are encouraged to continue to update their knowledge and maintain contact with those engaged in research on internal fixation through periodic participation in such courses.

Boston and Philadelphia   Gustave E. Fackelman
October 1981   David M. Nunamaker

Table of Contents

Part I

Part I

Chapter 1. Basic Principles of Fracture Treatment

The basic philosophy of the ASIF technique is functional fracture treatment provided by stable internal fixation and early mobilization of the joints with partial and then full weight bearing. Stable internal fixation is achieved through accurate anatomic reduction and interfragmentary compression of the bone fragments so that the injured bone itself transmits and supports weight-bearing loads. Exact anatomic reduction can be accomplished with screws alone or with screws and one or more plates. The intimate contact between the reduced fragments, necessary for stability of the reduced fractures, can be achieved with interfragmentary compression. Complete reconstruction of the bone is absolutely necessary in order to transfer weight-bearing loads through the bone, thus sparing the relatively weak implant (Fig. 1.1a). This basic premise allows successful fracture treatment in a large animal, such as the horse, without the use of implants that might overpower the bone. Any inability to transmit loads across the fracture site will result in implant deformation (Fig. 1.1b) and/or failure of the implant (Fig. 1.1c).

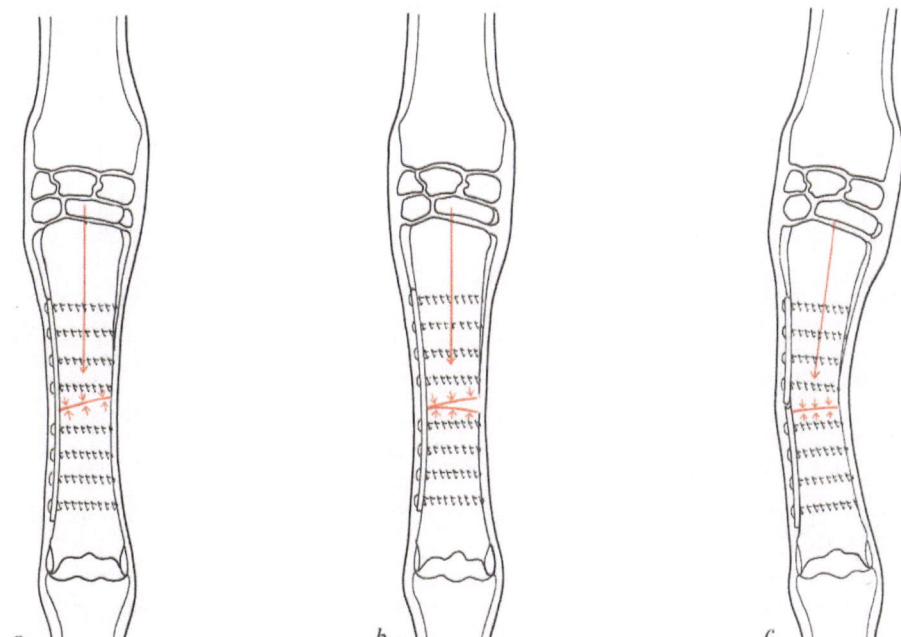

Fig. 1.1 a–c. *a* Load transmission across the fracture line after anatomic reduction with resultant stability. *b* Any inability to transmit loads across the fracture site will result in implant deformation. *c* Persistent cyclic deformation will result in implant failure.

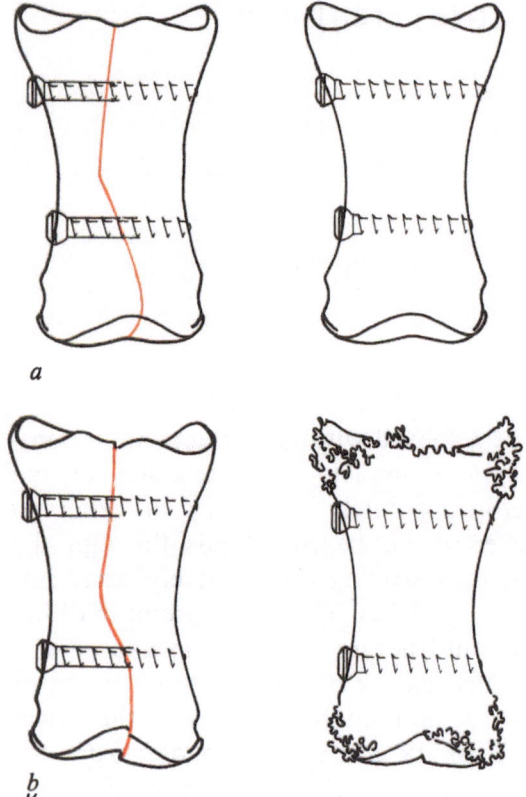

Fig. 1.2 a, b. *a* The potential good result obtained with perfect anatomic reduction. *b* The bad result after inadequate reduction.

1.1 Accurate Reduction of the Fracture Fragments

Normal joint function can be maintained only if fractures through articular surfaces are accurately and anatomically reduced and stabilized so that congruence of the joint surfaces is maintained (Fig. 1.2a). Even a small step in the joint surface will lead to a degenerative joint with proliferative, peri-articular changes that may preclude a functional recovery (Fig. 1.2b). Such demanding surgery usually requires visualization of the fracture and the joint surface and new or more radical surgical exposures than have

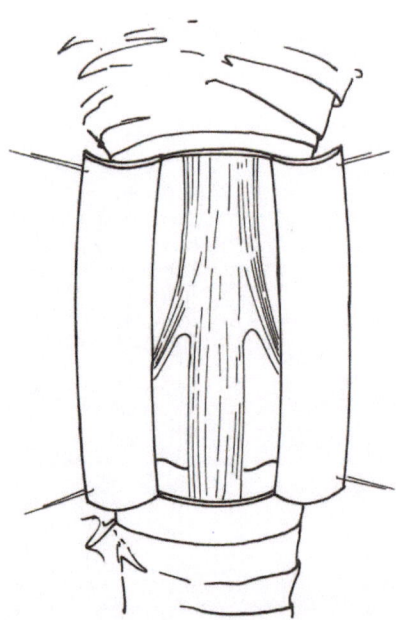

Fig. 1.3. Wide exposure of a first phalangeal fracture allows the adequate visualization of the fracture necessary for its repair.

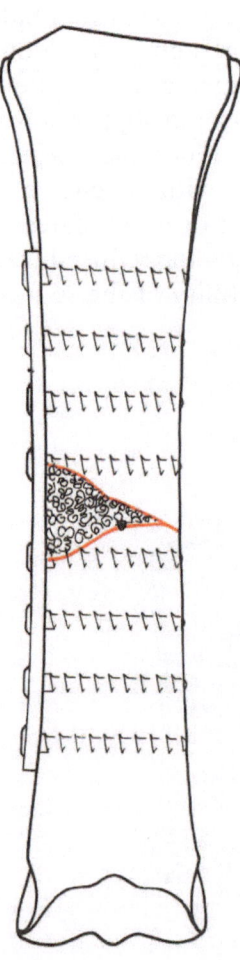

Fig. 1.4. A cancellous bone graft is used to form a bridge across any gap caused by comminution of the fracture. Note the placement of the plate over the area of comminution to maintain stability.

been advocated in the past (Fig. 1.3). Comminution, which plays such a great role in the equine shaft fractures, emphasizes the need for anatomic reduction of the fragments with the use of cancellous bone grafts. Direct continuity must be maintained across the fracture site, either by using the animal's own cortical bone or with a mass of cancellous bone that can eventually form a solid bridge (Fig. 1.4). The plate is placed over the area of comminution to maintain stability. Whenever cancellous bone is used to cause the development of a buttress across a bony defect, weight bearing must be delayed. Full, immediate weight bearing in such cases will lead to catastrophic failure of the reduction and therefore of the internal fixation. In the horse, external fixation is necessary to prevent weight bearing, and full functional treatment is delayed until the bone-plate composite is capable of full weight support. Only when this stage is reached can mobilization of the associated joints begin. This present drawback of fracture treatment in the horse awaits further developments in operative techniques as well as in postoperative management.

1.2 Stable Internal Fixation

The heart of the ASIF system consists of achieving fixation by means of interfragmentary compression. Interfragmentary compression causes high frictional forces at the fracture surfaces, and these forces confer stability. Compression can be extended across the fracture site by the use of screws alone (Fig. 1.5a) or, as in the case of a transverse fracture, axial interfragmentary compression may be achieved by a combination of screws and a plate (Fig. 1.5b). Many times, reconstruction of a fracture in the horse requires both axial compression, applied through the use of a plate in combination with screws, and interfragmentary compression achieved by using screws alone (Fig. 1.5c).

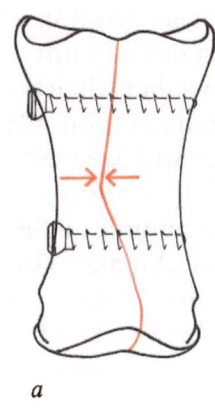

a

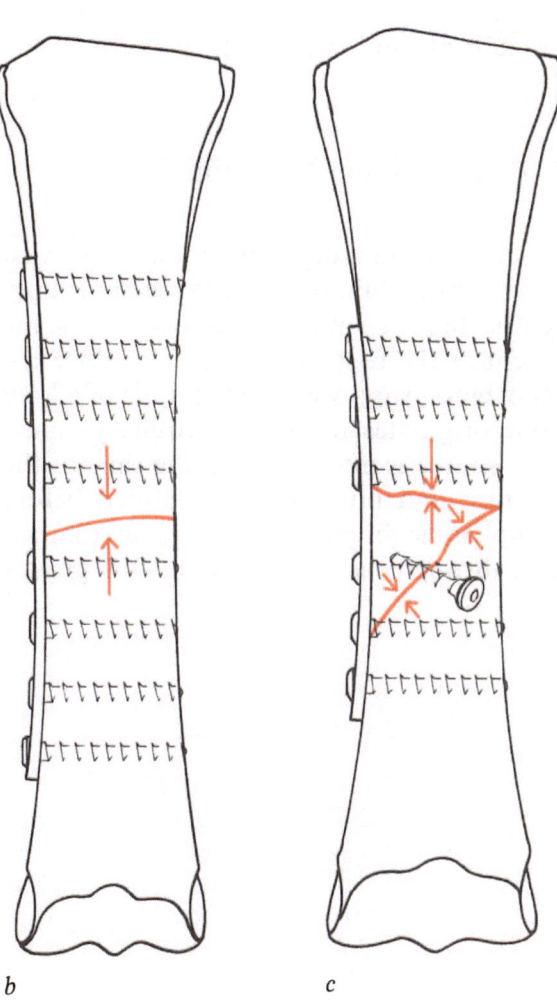

b   *c*

Fig. 1.5 a–c. *a* Sagittal first phalangeal fracture with screws providing interfragmentary compression. *b* A plate applied to the reduced fracture provides axial compression. *c* A combination of plate axial compression and interfragmentary screw compression in a comminuted fracture.

In stable internal fixation, the emphasis should be placed on the word "stable," since it has been shown that when bone fragments are approximated anatomically, subsequent motion interferes with fracture union. Therefore, it is very important for the surgeon to prevent relative motion at the fracture site when using this technique. This is not to say that fracture healing never occurs when there is motion at the fracture site, because it surely does, as demonstrated time and again with the use of casts and splints in many species. The key to this apparent discrepancy may lie in the distance between the ends of the fracture fragments in relationship to the amount of motion present.

1.3 Soft-Tissue Problems

Fracture healing depends on adequate vascularization of the bone. The vascular supply to the bone is always destroyed to some extent at the time of the fracture, since the main blood supply to the diaphysis of a long bone originates from the medullary canal. This source is interrupted at the time of the fracture and must be reconstituted before complete healing can occur. Revascularization through the medullary canal is greatly hastened by stable internal fixation, using compression techniques. The periosteal blood supply, however, becomes relatively more important before reconstitution of the medullary supply occurs. The periosteal blood comes from the surrounding soft tissues. In most equine fractures a great amount of energy is expended into the soft tissues at the time of the fracture. This explosion of the bone into the soft tissues may cause immediate disruption of the periosteal blood supply of the bone. Therefore, even before any surgical intervention, there is usually a great deal of damage already present around the fracture site, which may be the cause of significant postoperative complications, such as wound dehiscence, superficial and deep wound infections, and osteomyelitis. The risk of complications because of soft tissue injury must be weighed heavily before making a decision about open reduction and internal fixation. If surgery is indicated, it is of the utmost importance to maintain all remaining vascularity to the fractured bone. Some internal fixations may be achieved through stab incisions using fluoroscopic control. This procedure is usually accomplished in non-displaced fractures or in easily reduced simple fractures (Fig. 1.6). The soft tissues are protected during the internal fixation by using different drill

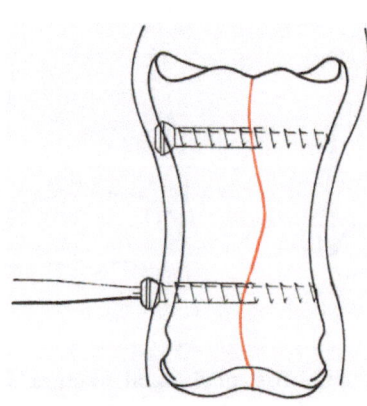

Fig. 1.6. Stab incisions can be used in non-displaced fractures for insertion of screws to minimize surgical soft-tissue injury.

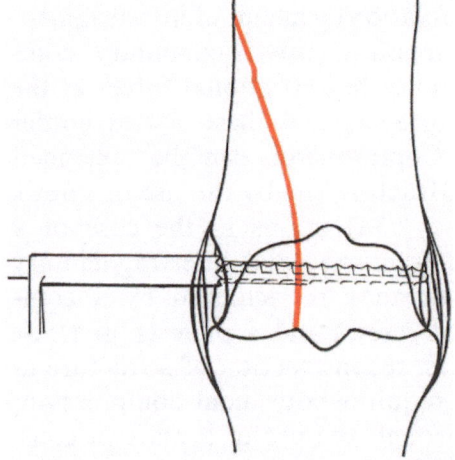

Fig. 1.7. Drill and tap guides are necessary to protect the soft tissues.

6

guides and tap sleeves (Fig. 1.7). At other times, wide exposures are necessary to reduce and stabilize badly comminuted fractures adequately. The apparent contradiction then exists between the preservation and protection of the soft tissues and the exposure necessary to perform proper anatomic reduction and internal fixation. The relatively high infection rate that accompanies equine long-bone fracture fixation is most likely related to the vascularity problem caused by high-energy fractures as they occur in the horse. In the horse, the limitation of other alternatives to internal fixation often necessitates taking this risk. No easy, quick solution can be given to circumvent this problem. Experience with other animal species lends little help, since this problem seems to be unique to the horse. Each surgeon's soft tissue handling technique will in great measure determine that individual's own limitations.

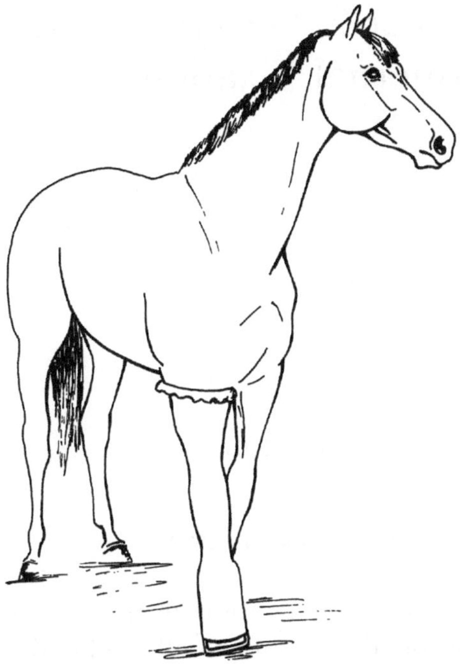

Fig. 1.8. A forelimb fracture is immobilized in a fiberglass cast with walking bar during the early postoperative period.

1.4 Early Return to Full Function

As previously stated, the purpose of internal fixation is to provide functional fracture treatment. This means that early weight bearing and a return of complete joint function and mobility in the absence of pain are the goals. In small animals, immediate full weight bearing can usually be achieved by restricting the patient to a small area. In large animals, immediate full weight bearing can lead to catastrophic failure of the implant, especially in comminuted fractures where there is no direct bridge or bone contact across the fracture site. In these cases, external fixation is necessary at least during the recovery phase and often for a period of time following recovery to allow the bone-plate composite to become strong enough for full, unprotected weight bearing

as shown in Fig. 1.8 in which a forelimb fracture has been immobilized in a fiberglass cast with walking bar during the early postoperative period. During this time, joint mobility is sacrificed to protect the implant and the attached bone from failure.

Although this represents a compromise with theoretical considerations, it accurately describes the state of the art and awaits further developments in surgical technique and postoperative care.

References

Perren, SM: Physical and biological aspects of fracture healing with special reference to internal fixation. Clinical Orthop. **138**, (1979): 175

Chapter 2. General Techniques and Biomechanics of Internal Fixation

2.1 Screw Fixation

2.1.1 Drilling Holes in Bone

Proper internal fixation using screws depends on the quality of the implants, the quality of the bone, and the technique of assembly. Although there is little we can do about the quality of bone, the technique of drilling a hole into the bone can have a profound effect on the success of the internal fixation. Therefore, it is important to be able to drill a hole properly. Since equine bone is very hard, drilling a hole through this type of bone may pose problems that are usually not encountered when drilling holes in bones of animals of other species.

Drill holes in bone should be round. Drill bit wobble during the drilling cycle produces oval holes, removing bone that would otherwise be present to support the screw. Drill guides are designed to help control the quality of a drill hole and to prevent drill bit wobble. Power drills allow a more controlled drill hole than do hand-powered braces. The power drill also helps prevent operator fatigue during long surgical procedures.

Another reason for drill wobble has to do with the drilling of crooked holes (Fig. 2.1a). The drill bit first penetrates the convex surface of the outer cortex (*cis* cortex) and then enters into the marrow cavity. If direct engagement of the drill bit is not made in the inner concave surface of the opposite cortex (*trans* cortex), the point of the drill bit will "walk" down the inclined plane until it engages somewhere in the *trans* cortex and then drills through it. If this occurs, the drill bit bends and the drill begins to wobble. A hole made in this manner will not be straight, and insertion of a screw into this hole may result in a weakened screw due to repeated plastic deformation during insertion.

If drill wobble occurs during the drilling cycle, the drill should be retracted and then advanced very slowly until engagement of the drill bit with the *trans* cortex occurs. At this point, full pressure can be exerted

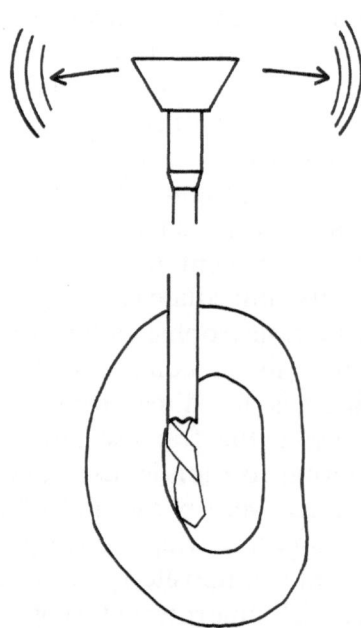

Fig. 2.1 a. Power drill wobble may be caused by the inability of the drill bit to engage in the *trans* cortex thus drilling a crooked hole.

against the bone and the hole drilled in a normal fashion.

The generation of heat during the drilling cycle can be reduced by increasing the cutting rate. The cutting rate depends on the cutting characteristics of the drill bit, as well as the force exerted on it. Minimizing frictional forces by lubrication can also improve the cutting rate (Fig. 2.1b). Controlling heat directly by cooling with irrigation solution is impractical. Fluid volumes in excess of 300 ml/min must be used to influence the temperature of the bone. Heat is reduced secondarily by improving lubrication and facilitating removal of debris. Although low-speed drills have been advocated in orthopedic surgery to reduce heat generation, the experimental literature does not indicate the superiority of any particular drilling speed. The real control that the surgeon exerts over the rate of drilling holes into bone is the force directed down the shaft of the drill. In general, in bone, the greater the force exerted, the faster the drilling will be and the less heat will be generated. Certainly, care must be taken not to overload the equipment and cause breakage of the drill bit or damage to the soft tissue when the drill bit penetrates the *trans* cortex.

Careful maintenance of a drill bit will also improve its continued performance. Normally, unless the drill bit strikes metal objects, it will drill through more than one meter of bone before it needs sharpening. The bone cuttings, also called swath material, must be removed from the cutting site. This swath material contains much of the heat generated in the bone during the drilling cycle and must pass up the flutes of the drill bit to be removed at the surface (Fig. 2.2). When using drill guides, this material is often trapped and cannot be removed. It packs into the flutes and successfully halts all cutting action of the drill bit, resulting in great increases in heat production. Therefore, periodic cleaning of the drill bit is necessary. The lands of the drill bit are designed so that lubricant can be directed behind them toward the tip of the drill to reduce friction. Thus, a circulation system is formed to

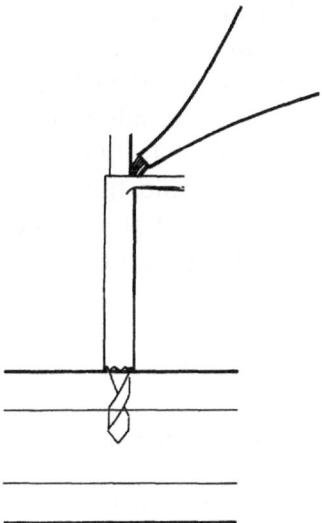

Fig. 2.1b. Irrigation during drilling is useful to decrease friction and thereby increase drilling rate.

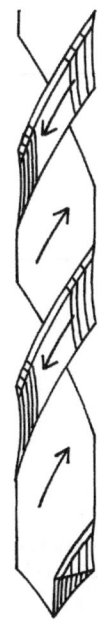

Fig. 2.2. The irrigation solution passes down the drill bit behind the lands and is removed with the swath material in the flutes, creating a circulation system that reduces friction and thus allows the drill bit to cut more efficiently.

introduce lubricant (in this case saline) to the drilling point and. then remove it with the swath material in the drill flutes. This reduces friction and thus allows the drill bit to cut more efficiently. Drill bits that are bent should be replaced, and those that are dull should be discarded or sharpened. Optimal drilling rates with presently available drill bits are about 1 mm/s. Lower rates may result in excessive heating of the bone.

2.1.2 Types of Screws

There are two basic types of screws used in bone: cancellous and cortical.

Table 2.1. Screw Sizes with Appropriate Drill Bits and Taps (Sizes in mm)

Outside diameter of screw	Screw tap size	Core diameter of screw	Drill bit Pilot hole	Gliding hole
1.5 Cortical	1.5	1.0	1.1	1.5
2.0 Cortical	2.0	1.3	1.5	2.0
2.7 Cortical	2.7	1.9	2.0	2.7
3.5[a]	3.5	1.9	2.0	3.5
3.5[b] Cortical	3.5	2.4	2.5	3.5
4.0 Small Cancellous	3.5[c]	1.9	2.0	Cancellous screw N/A[e]
4.5 Cortical	4.5	3.0	3.2	4.5
5.5[d] Cortical	5.5			5.5
6.5 Large cancellous	6.5	3.0	3.2 3.6 in hard bone	Cancellous screw N/A 4.5 mm for guiding hole in hard bone if necessary

[a] This screw has been a standard ASIF screw for many years and has cancellous bone screw characteristics.

[b] This 3.5 mm screw is relatively new and has an increased core diameter for improved strength and a finer cortical thread that holds better in hard bone. Because of its increased diameter, it is recommended by the authors for equine applications. This screw has typical cortical bone screw characteristics.

[c] The tap for the 4.0 small cancellous screw is 3.5 mm and is designed so that the 4.0 mm small cancellous screw will cut the additional 0.5 mm of thread during its insertion into soft cancellous bone. This screw therefore is for use in soft cancellous bone only.

[d] This 5.5 mm screw has, until now, been purely an experimental screw. Initial tests have shown it to be about twice as strong in both breaking strength and in axial compression generation as the standard 4.5 mm screw.

[e] N/A = not applicable.

a) Cancellous Screws

The cancellous screw (Fig. 2.3 a) is partially threaded and produces interfragmentary compression using a single-diameter drill bit and tap to allow the screw to obtain purchase only at its distal threaded end (Table 2.1). In this way, the proximal part of the screw glides through the *cis* cortex, and the seating of the head of the screw in the bone allows the interfragmentary compression to occur. The threaded portion of the screw when seated must not cross the fracture line, since this would prevent interfragmentary compression (Fig.2.3 b). The cancellous screw is available in two diameters, with the large 6.5 mm cancellous screw available in two different threaded lengths (16 and 32 mm).

The cancellous screw should be used in soft cancellous bone where a cortical screw would not hold. This screw is not indicated for hard cancellous bone or in cortical bone for the purpose of obtaining better fixation. Normally, this screw would rarely be used in the horse; its use is indicated only to obtain interfragmentary compression when the cortical screw has stripped; to obtain purchase, in some cases, in the proximal fragment of an olecranon fracture; or in osteoporotic bone, which may be present in young animals for various reasons. There are two basic reasons for the limitation of its use: 1) The cancellous screw is partially threaded, and if used in equine cortical bone, it may be impossible to remove after healing has taken place. This is due to the fact that bone will grow around the smooth shaft of the proximal end of the screw and prevent the screw from cutting its threads through this bone during attempts to remove it. If an effort is made to remove this screw after healing has occurred, the screw will break, leaving the threaded portion embedded in the bone. 2) The weak point of any partially threaded screw lies at the junction between the shaft and its threads. In

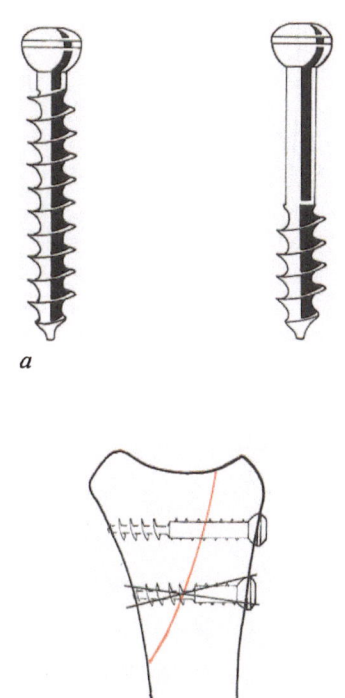

a

b

Fig. 2.3 a, b. *a* The large cancellous screws come in two sizes according to the length of the threaded portion. *b* If the use of a cancellous screw should be necessary, care must be taken to allow for interfragmentary compression. (See text.)

hard equine bone, the screw may break here during insertion. Table 2.1 shows that two different drill bit diameters are recommended. In normal equine cancellous bone (hard bone) the 3.6 mm drill bit is preferred. Since the shaft of the large cancellous screw is 4.5 mm in diameter, it reduces the effort of inserting this screw even after the use of the 6.5 mm tap. In normal equine cortical bone, the 4.5 mm drill is needed to drill a clearance hole for the shaft. If this is necessary, a cortical screw should be used instead of the cancellous one.

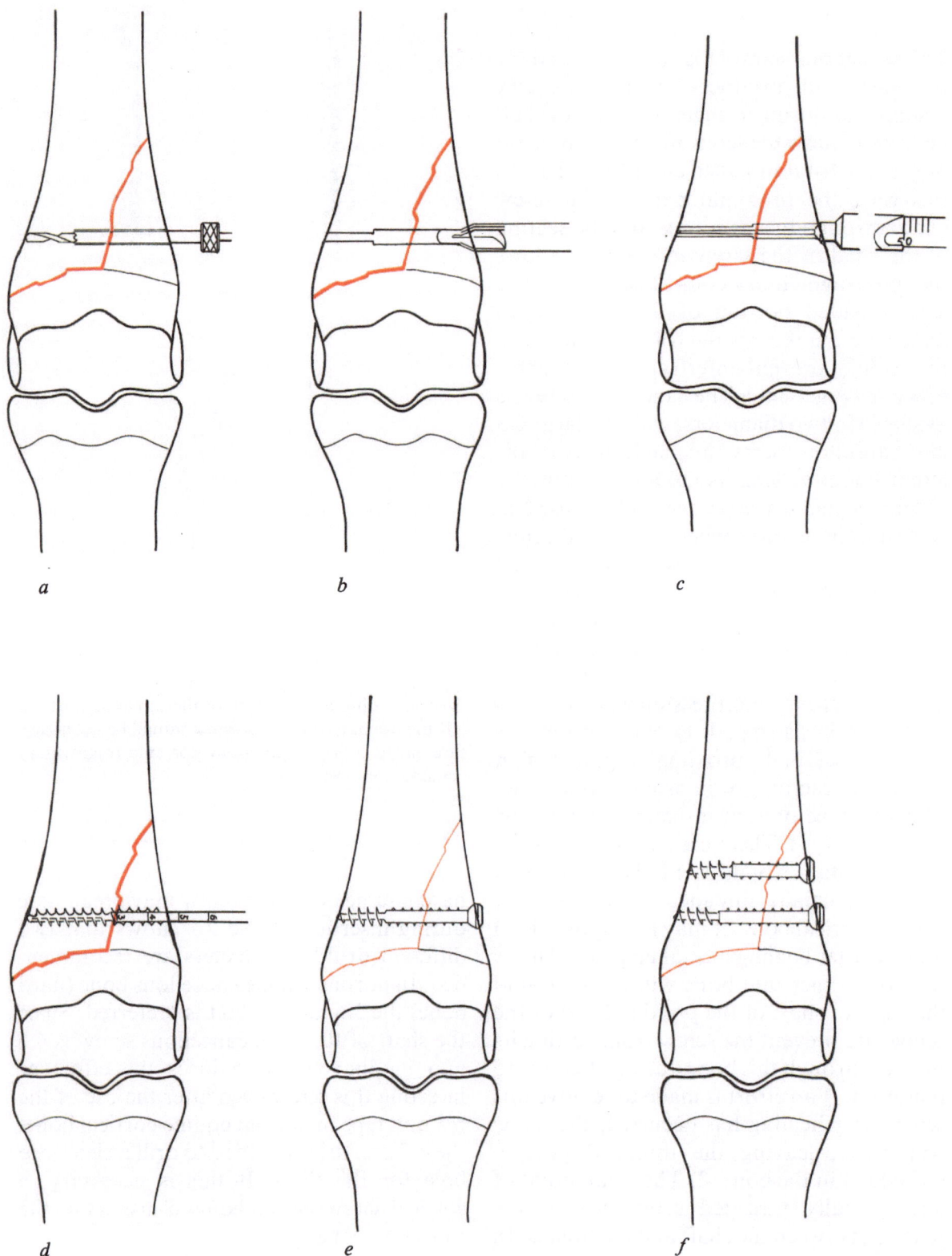

Fig. 2.4 a–f. Technique for cancellous screw insertion. *a* A hole is drilled through both cortices. *b* Use of the countersink. *c* Measuring for screw length with the depth gauge. *d* Tapping the pilot hole and checking for depth with the cancellous tap. *e* Insertion and tightening of the first cancellous screw. *f* Two cancellous screws inserted and uniformly tightened

The *technique of insertion* is shown in Figure 2.4. After reduction of the fracture fragments with a bone-holding forceps or other device, a hole of the proper dimension is drilled through both cortices (Fig. 2.4a). The countersink is used to provide a seat for the cancellous screw head (Fig. 2.4b), and the hole is measured using the depth gauge (Fig. 2.4c). Next, the proper size tap is used to cut the thread in the bone; a depth gauge is included on the large 6.5 mm cancellous tap so that the length of the screw may be checked at the time of tapping (Fig. 2.4d). The tap should turn easily and be backed off periodically to remove the swath material from the cutting threads. The usual routine is two half-turns forward then one quarter-turn back. This routine varies with the density of the bone, but the tap should never be advanced with great force since it can break and is difficult to remove. The proper size screw is then inserted and tightened (Fig. 2.4e). In general, all screws should be tightened uniformly (Fig. 2.4f). The degree of force necessary is difficult to describe, but it is somewhere between the limits of tightening as much as possible with fingers alone (Fig. 2.5a) and moderately strong tightening using the palm of the hand on the screwdriver handle (Fig. 2.5b). This translates into a torque of between 400 and 600 Newton-cm. Whenever a cortical screw has failed, it is only necessary to use the proper size cancellous tap in the failed screw hole and then insert and tighten the screw. Occasionally in *very* soft bone it is even possible to insert the cancellous screw into the failed cortical screw hole without tapping.

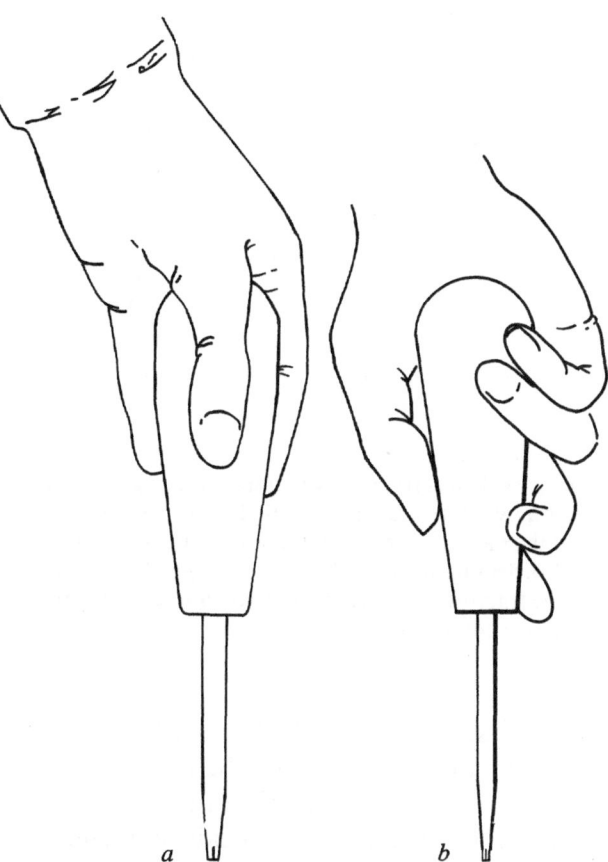

Fig. 2.5 a, b. *a* Tightening with the screwdriver is shown, using fingers alone. *b* Here the palm of the hand is added to give more power to the tightening procedure.

b) Cortical Screws

A cortical screw (Fig. 2.6) is completely threaded and produces interfragmentary compression using a large gliding hole in the *cis* cortex and a narrow threaded (pilot) hole in the *trans* cortex (Fig. 2.7a). The ASIF

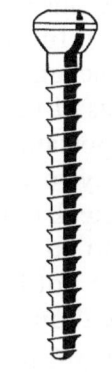

Fig. 2.6. A fully threaded cortical screw.

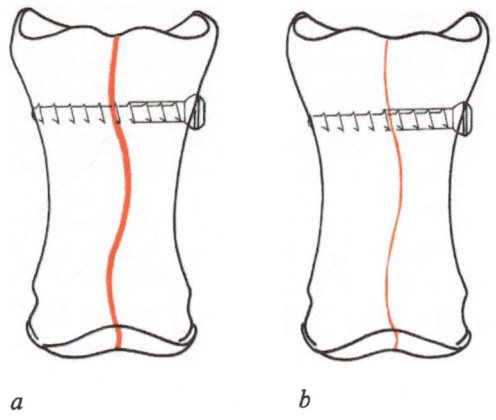

a   *b*

Fig. 2.7 a, b. *a* A fracture is compressed using a cortical lag screw. Note the large gliding hole in the *cis* cortex and the narrow threaded pilot hole in the *trans* cortex. *b* Overdrilling through the endosteal bone all the way to the fracture site is necessary to obtain real interfragmentary compression.

cortical screws are available in a wide variety of sizes (Table 2.1), and their use as lag screws necessitates the utilization of a large drill bit equivalent to the outside diameter of the screw thread to provide the gliding hole through the *cis* cortex, and a smaller drill bit, equivalent to the approximate core diameter of the screw, to drill the smaller hole that will be threaded in the *trans* cortex. In this way, the fully threaded cortical screw can be used as a lag screw just like the cancellous screw. Here again, as with the cancellous lag screw, the threads of the screw find purchase only in one cortex (*trans* cortex) and do not engage bone on the opposite side of the fracture line (*cis* cortex) (Fig. 2.7). In the horse, there is usually a considerable amount of cancellous bone in the diaphysis of many of the bones. Therefore, it is important that the gliding hole goes all the way to the fracture plane through any endosteal bone that may be present. It is better to go a little too far with the gliding hole than not far enough. If the screw is inserted without overdrilling, the screw will hold the fragments apart, the production of callus is encouraged, and the fixation will probably fail.

In the horse, cortical screws should be used in cortical and hard cancellous bone. Since equine bone generally is very hard, there are few reasons for not using cortical lag screws. If by chance the bone fails, i.e., the screw strips on insertion, a larger diameter cortical or cancellous screw may be used in the same screw hole. Therefore, when in doubt regarding the type of screw to use, try the cortical screw first with the possibility of the cancellous screw as a replacement should stripping occur on insertion. Since cortical screws are fully threaded, they are more easily removed than cancellous screws, and their fully threaded form makes them uniformly strong so that failure along the shaft of the screw during insertion is quite uncommon.

The *technique of insertion* is shown in Figure 2.8. After reduction of the fracture fragments with a bone-holding forceps, a C-clamp, or other device, a large gliding hole is drilled through the *cis* cortex and, if necessary, through the endosteal cancellous bone to the fracture site (Fig. 2.8a). A drill insert is placed into this hole and pushed through until it engages the fracture line or opposite *trans* cortex. This drill insert has the same outside diameter as the gliding hole that was previously drilled and an inner diameter which will accept the drill bit for the pilot hole in the *trans* cortex. The insert functions to center the pilot hole precisely in relation to the gliding hole (Fig. 2.8b). The hole in the *trans* cortex is then drilled with the proper size drill bit and, thereafter, the drill bit and the insert are removed. A countersink is used to provide a seat for the head of the cortical screw (Fig. 2.8c), and the hole is then measured with the depth gauge (Fig. 2.8d). It is important to turn the countersink completely in a 360° arc to achieve a smooth surface on which the screw head will be seated.

The cortical tap is introduced into the hole, and threads are cut in the bone (Fig. 2.8e). The tap is advanced two half-turns and then backed off one quarter-turn to clean the swath material from the threads of the tap. It is important that the tap moves easily. If binding occurs, further advancement should cease immediately since it may cause breakage of the instrument. Frequent cleaning is necessary to remove the swath material from the longitudinal grooves of the tap. After the threads have been satisfactorily cut, a screw of the proper length is inserted and tightened (Fig. 2.8f). Saline or balanced electrolyte solution, added as a lubricant during drilling (Fig. 2.9a) and tapping (Fig. 2.9b) of the hole as well as at the time of insertion of the screw (Fig. 2.9c), will reduce

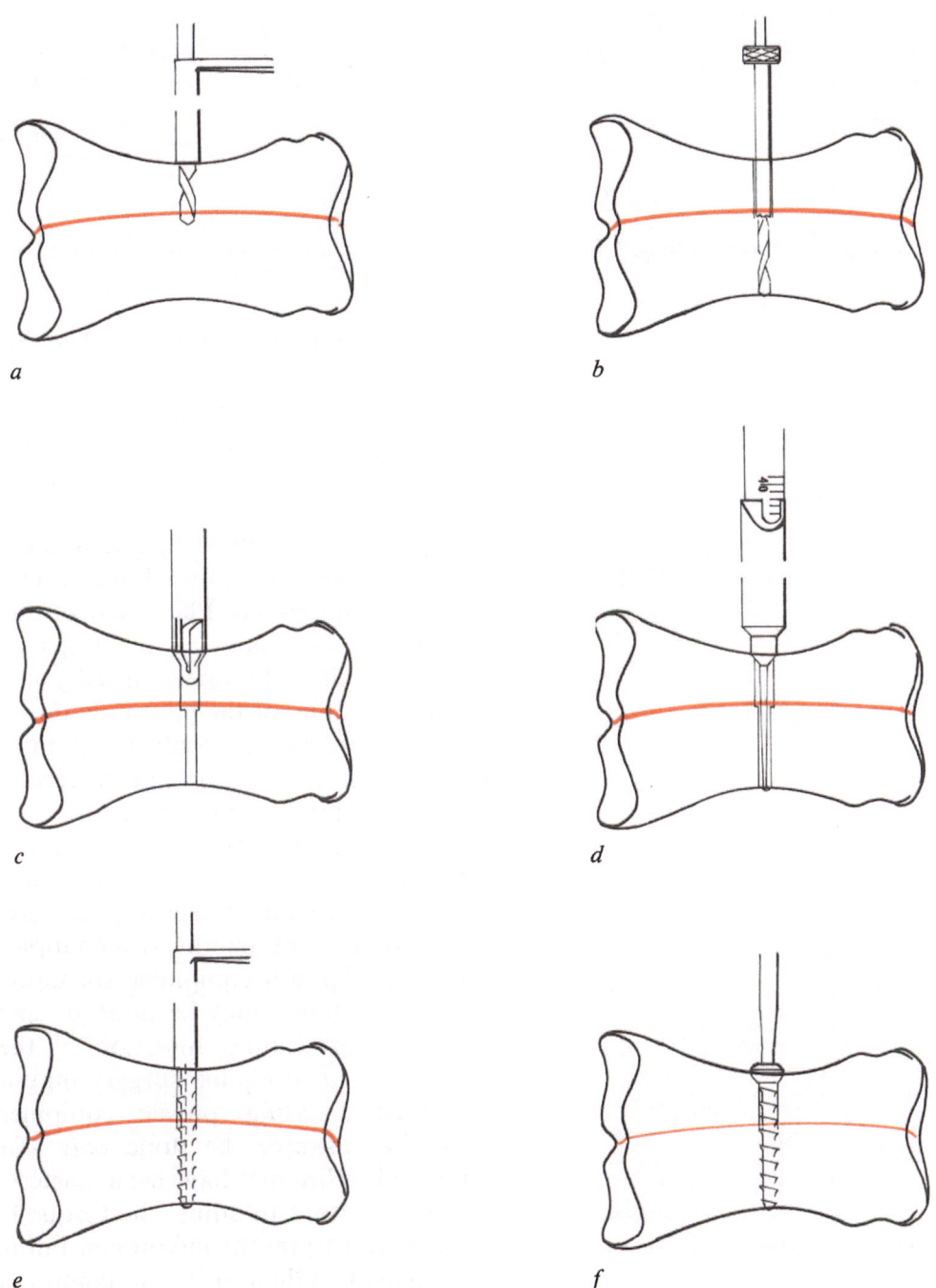

Fig. 2.8 a–f. Technique of cortical screw insertion. *a* Drilling the gliding hole. *b* Positioning the drill guide insert and drilling the pilot hole. *c* Use of the countersink. *d* Measuring for screw length with the depth gauge. *e* Tapping. *f* Inserting and tightening the cortical screw.

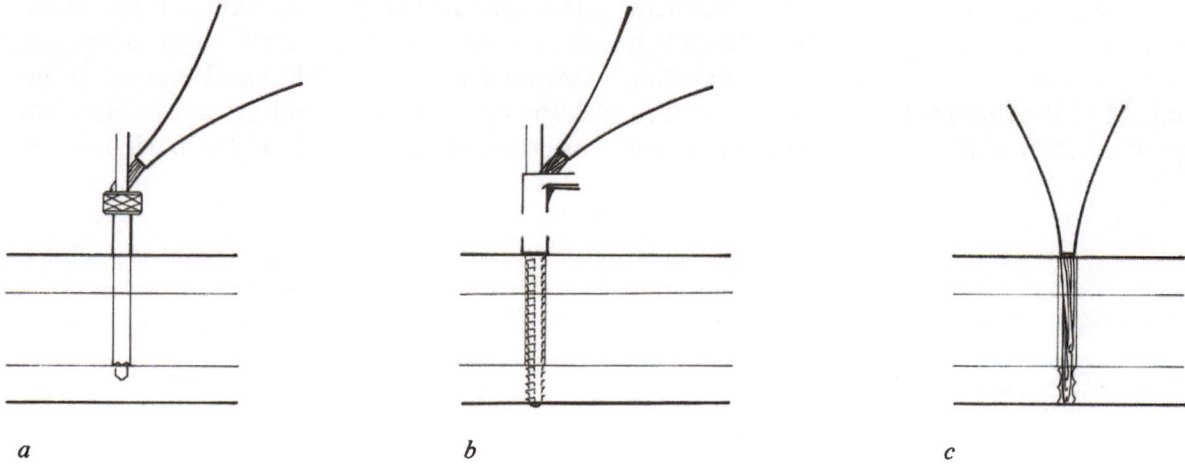

Fig. 2.9 a–c. *a* Irrigation during drilling. *b* Irrigation during tapping. *c* Irrigation prior to inserting the screw.

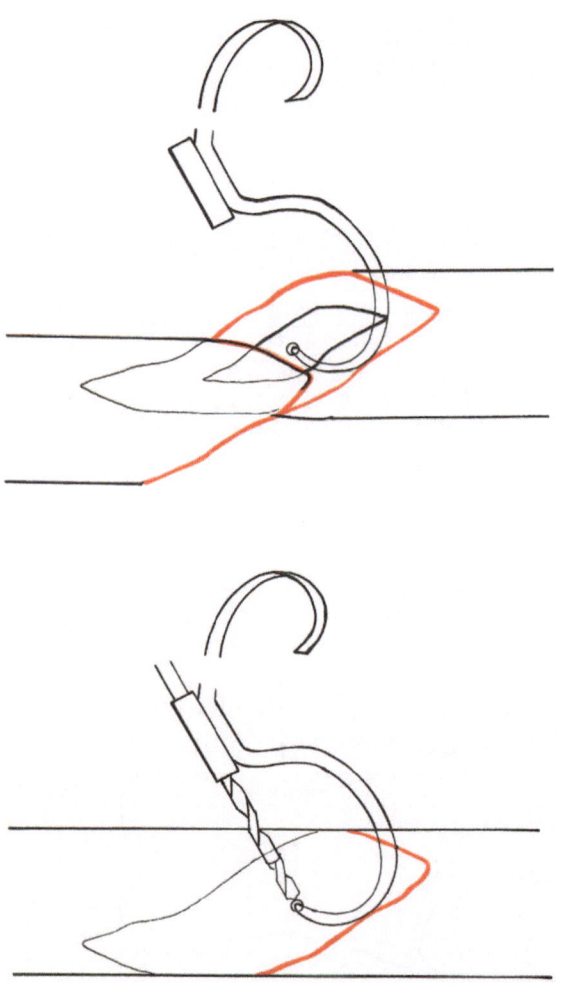

Fig. 2.10. The use of the hooked drill guide allows the placement of the pilot hole before reduction of the fragments to be sure of the accurate placement of the hole.

the friction necessary to complete the internal fixation.

Occasionally, because of a narrow posterior spike on the *trans* cortex, it is necessary to drill the *trans* cortex first and then reduce the fracture. Here, the hooked drill guide (Fig. 2.10) will allow the gliding hole to be placed after reduction of the fracture has been accomplished. Placement of the screw is then done following the steps outlined above. This technique is usually necessary only if drilling of the pilot hole through the drill insert could result in inappropriate placement; for instance, in the fracture line or out of the fracture fragment.

Although the power drill is recommended for drilling holes in bone, tapping of the screw thread and insertion of the screws are usually done by hand. Power tapping, i.e., the use of power equipment for tapping the thread in bone, may be done to speed the surgical procedure. Insertion of the long screws used in equine surgery may also be performed using power equipment. It should, however, be done *only* after the manual techniques have been mastered, and it is important to adjust the torque level of the drill, to prevent instrument failure (tap breakage). When using a compressed-air system, this can be easily done by decreasing the pressure available to the drill. The ASIF small drill also has an instant reversing

16

trigger which allows the backing up of the tap for cleaning purposes and periodic reversal during the tapping procedure to remove the swath material from the cutting edges of the tap, as has been described for the manual tapping procedure. When using this method for insertion of screws, manual tightening should be performed on every screw after its insertion.

2.1.3 Position of the Screws

The position of the screw relative to the fracture site is very important. In general, stability is achieved across fracture surfaces by normal forces, i.e., forces perpendicular to the fracture plane (Fig. 2.11a). Shearing forces (forces parallel to the fracture plane) will potentially cause sliding and instability (Fig. 2.11b). Therefore, to insure stability through high frictional forces, screw placement should result in high normal forces without shearing forces. In spiral fractures, this is accomplished by following the spiral with the interfragmentary screws to maximize the normal forces in both the longitudinal (Fig. 2.12a) and the transverse planes (Fig. 2.12b).

The problem becomes more complicated when dealing with the longitudinal plane. Here, high normal forces are desired, but in addition to the loading of the bone by the screw (interfragmentary compression), there is an axial loading of the bone by the weight of the animal, which will change the resultant load on the fracture plane. Therefore, it is important to balance the load and the direction of the force of the screw so that they interact with the axial load due to the weight of the animal, resulting in forces exerted at the fracture plane which are normal to it. On the basis of theoretical considerations and practical experience, fractures in the horse that have a surface length greater than twice the width of the bone, require screws inserted perpendicular to the long axis of the bone. This would include condylar fractures of the third metacarpal bone and longitudinal fractures of the first phalanx.

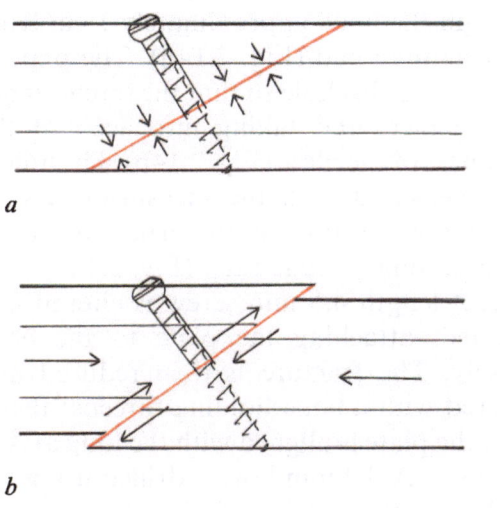

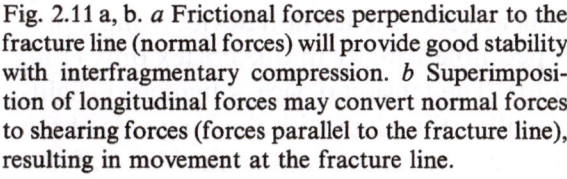

Fig. 2.11 a, b. a Frictional forces perpendicular to the fracture line (normal forces) will provide good stability with interfragmentary compression. b Superimposition of longitudinal forces may convert normal forces to shearing forces (forces parallel to the fracture line), resulting in movement at the fracture line.

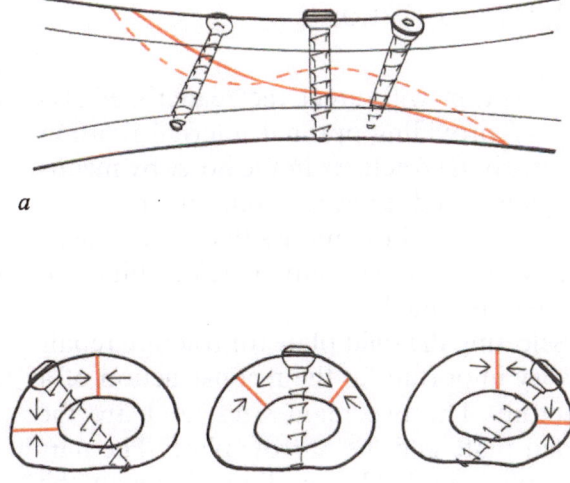

Fig. 2.12 a, b. Placement of the screw maximizes the normal forces in both the longitudinal and transverse plane.

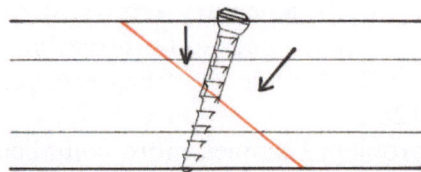

Fig. 2.13. This interfragmentary screw is placed in a compromise position between perpendicular to the fracture site and perpendicular to the long axis of the bone.

Fracture lines that are less than twice the width of the bone should be repaired by screws placed in a compromise position between perpendicular to the fracture plane and perpendicular to the long axis of the bone (Fig. 2.13). Rarely, and only if other interfragmentary screws are used, should a screw be placed perpendicular to the fracture plane in the horse. The potential effect of weight bearing on the fracture could be disastrous.

In all cases, the resultant force carried across the fracture surface should be a normal one.

2.2 Plate Fixation

This section will direct the reader's efforts toward providing optimal internal fixation of long-bone fractures in the horse by means of plates and screws. Concepts of plate application and techniques that may be used in any area and with any plate combination will be presented.

Selecting the right plate for fracture repair is very important in the reconstruction of a fracture. The two main sizes used are the broad plate and the narrow plate. The narrow plate probably has limited use in the horse because of its low strength. It may be used in foals and occasionally in double plating (two plates on the same fracture). Choosing the right length of a plate represents another decision of much significance.

When applying the standard round-hole plate, the tension device must be attached to the end of it along the length of the bone; therefore, the plate chosen must be short enough to accommodate the tension device. In equine fractures in general, the bone is plated from end to end. One advantage of the dynamic compression plate is the ease with which a longer plate may be used.

2.2.1 Types of Plates

a) Round Hole Plate

The technique for applying the plate will be described using the standard round-hole ASIF plate (Fig. 2.14) and the dynamic compression plate (DCP) (Fig. 2.15) together with the standard 4.5 mm cortical screw. The technique for the other size screws and plates is the same, and the instrumentation is sized for these also. The correct drill bit and tap for each screw size can be found in Table 2.1.

After deciding on the proper plate (broad or narrow), determining the proper length of the plate, and contouring the plate to the fractured bone, a 3.2 mm hole is drilled through the bone approximately 1 cm from the fractured end (Fig. 2.14a). The plate is placed over this hole so that the screw length can be measured taking into account the thickness of the plate (Fig. 2.14b). The hole is first measured with the measuring device, then tapped through both cortices using the 4.5 mm long threaded tap (Fig. 2.14c). The correct length 4.5 mm screw is chosen and inserted, attaching the plate to the bone loosely. The fracture is then reduced and secured with a bone-holding forceps: thereafter the plate is aligned with the long axis of the bone. A 3.2 mm hole is drilled using the guide for the tension device, followed by application of the tension device using a pre-tapped hole usually in one cortex only (Fig. 2.14d). The tension device is tightened slightly to align the plate with the long axis of the bone and to approximate the ends of the

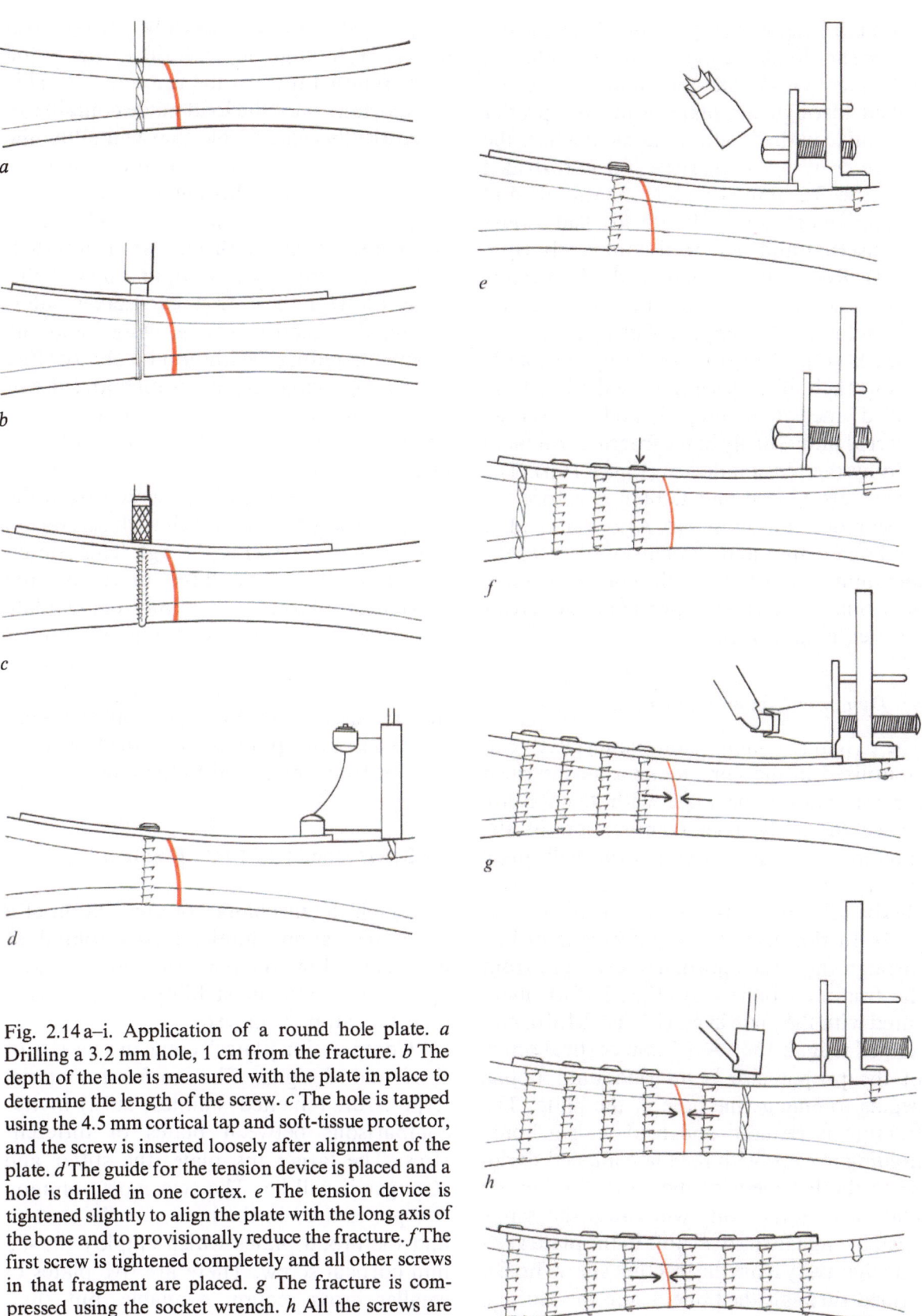

Fig. 2.14 a–i. Application of a round hole plate. *a* Drilling a 3.2 mm hole, 1 cm from the fracture. *b* The depth of the hole is measured with the plate in place to determine the length of the screw. *c* The hole is tapped using the 4.5 mm cortical tap and soft-tissue protector, and the screw is inserted loosely after alignment of the plate. *d* The guide for the tension device is placed and a hole is drilled in one cortex. *e* The tension device is tightened slightly to align the plate with the long axis of the bone and to provisionally reduce the fracture. *f* The first screw is tightened completely and all other screws in that fragment are placed. *g* The fracture is compressed using the socket wrench. *h* All the screws are now placed on this side of the fracture. *i* The tension device is removed and the remaining screws are placed.

fractured fragment (Fig. 2.14e). The tension device should not be tightened completely at this time. Next, the remaining holes are drilled through the plate, using the proper drill guide in the fracture fragment where the first screw was placed. These holes are drilled with the 3.2 mm drill bit, measured, and tapped as previously described. The screws are inserted and tightened completely (Fig. 2.14f). Remember to tighten the first screw that was loosely inserted. The tension device is then tightened completely using the socket wrench (Fig. 2.14g) followed by the open-end wrench, if necessary. Now the holes are drilled, measured, tapped, and the screws inserted individually in the fracture fragment held by the tension device (Fig. 2.14h). The screws are placed and tightened before the tension device is loosened. After removal of the bone clamp and the tension device, the remaining screw holes at the end of the plate are drilled, measured, tapped and the screws inserted (Fig. 2.14i).

b) Dynamic Compression Plate

The dynamic compression plate (DCP) can be utilized in the same manner as described for the round-hole plate with the tension device to apply axial compression to the fracture ends, using the neutral drill guide throughout the procedure. It can, however, also be used as a self-compressing plate (Fig. 2.15). In this case, a 3.2 mm hole is drilled through the bone approximately 1 cm from the fractured bone end (Fig. 2.15a), measured with the plate in place (Fig. 2.15b), and tapped (Fig. 2.15c). A 4.5 mm cortical screw of the proper size is inserted until it just begins to engage the hole in the plate. The fracture is reduced and held with a bone-holding forceps with the plate aligned parallel to the long axis of the bone. Sliding the plate across the bone will cause the screw head to engage the oval hole in the plate at its far edge away from the fracture site. A hole is drilled through the bone, using the 1.0 mm load guide in the screw hole nearest to the fracture site in the other fracture fragment

(Fig. 2.15d). This hole must be drilled using the *yellow* load guide, with the arrow of the guide pointed toward the fracture site. This is important since the load guide contains an eccentrically placed hole that will allow the screw being used to effect compression of the fractured bone ends through translocation of the plate. This hole is measured and tapped, and the screw of the proper size is inserted. The bone clamp is removed, and upon tightening both of these first two screws alternately, the fracture gap is closed and the fragments reduced with good stability (Fig. 2.15e). The remaining holes on both sides of the fracture may be drilled using the *green, neutral* drill guide (Fig. 2.15f). The holes are measured, tapped, and the screws inserted. Alternate tightening of the screws from the center outward, to insure that all screws are tight, is necessary (Fig. 2.15g). This should be repeated two or three times, as any movement of one screw may cause plate translocation, hence loosening of another screw. The central two screws that were used initially to create the axial compression of the fractured ends should be replaced with new ones at this point because the heads will be bent from the initial tightening.

2.2.2 Mechanics of Plate Fixation

Although the mechanics of application of a plate may seem simple, it is essential to understand how the plate functions, so that optimal strength and stability of the internal fixation can be achieved.

"Compression plates" come in a variety of sizes and designs. The uniform material (type 316L remelted stainless steel) invites comparisons between plates of different sizes. The larger the plate, the stiffer and stronger it will be. The two most common size plates used in the horse are the narrow and the broad plates which employ the 4.5 mm cortical screw. There are five plates of smaller cross section available, but since these are of little or no significance in the horse, they will not be discussed.

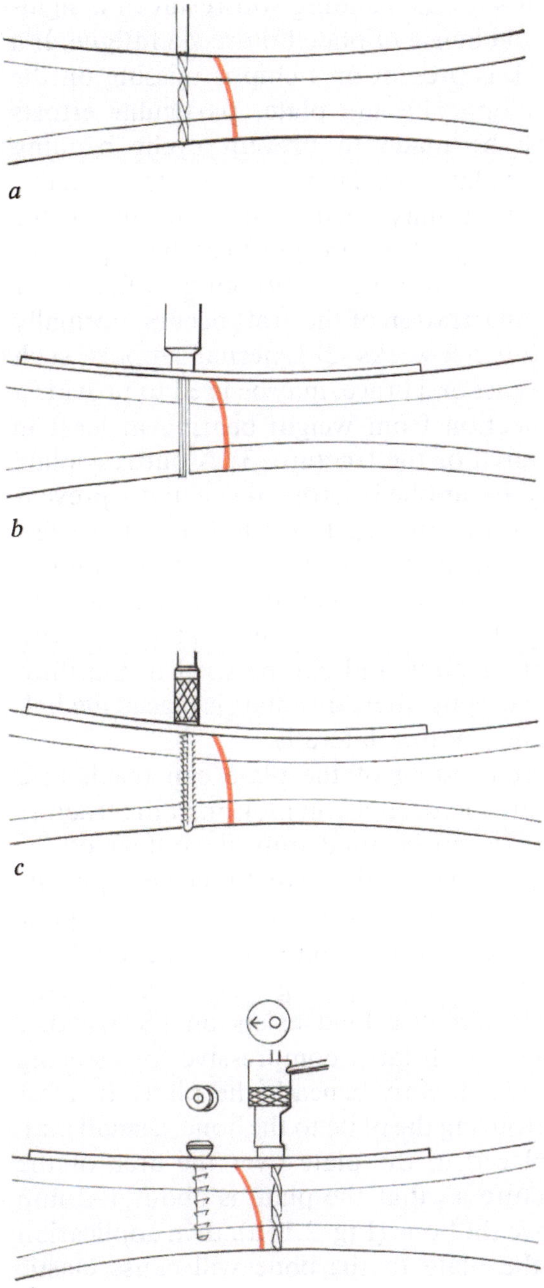

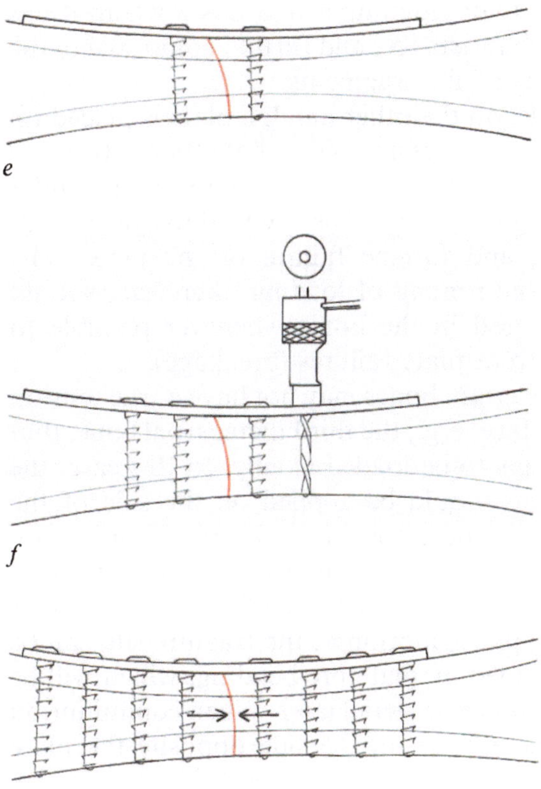

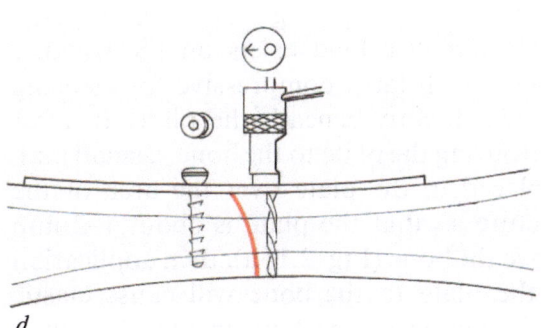

a

b

c

d

e

f

g

Fig. 2.15 a–g. Application of a dynamic compression plate. *a* Drilling a 3.2 mm hole, 1 cm from the fracture. *b* The depth of this hole is measured with the plate in place to determine the length of the screw. *c* The hole is tapped using the 4.5 mm cortical tap and soft-tissue protector, and the screw inserted loosely after alignment of the plate, until the head of the screw starts to engage the oval hole of the dynamic compression plate. *d* The plate is now displaced toward the fracture line and a hole is drilled through the plate using the 1.0 mm yellow load guide (eccentric hole). *e* Both screws are tightened alternately to approximate the edges of the fracture. *f* Additional screws on both sides of the fracture are then placed with the green neutral guide (hole in the center). *g* All the screws are tightened starting at the fracture site.

Plates used for internal fixation are strongest in tension and compression and weakest in bending. Plate fixations are also weak in torsion; however, this weakness is related not to the plate itself, but to its fasteners, the screws. Therefore, when using a "compression" plate, the objective is to place the plate on the tension side of the bone, i.e., the side of the bone which under physiological weight bearing conditions would normally subject it to mainly tensile forces. When this plate is applied under tension, forcing the ends of the bone in compression, a stable fixation is achieved. Normal weight bearing would then apply further tension (tension side of the bone) to the plate, loading it in a mode where it has high resistance, and further compressing the ends of the fragments.

If, on the other hand, a plate is placed on the compression side of the bone, bending stresses can be created in the plate under weight bearing. This can lead to cyclic bending and fatigue failure of the plate. The tension mode of loading, therefore, should be used in the horse whenever possible to prevent plate failures (breakage).

Certain bones may not have a true tension surface, e. g., the third metacarpal bone, that seems to be loaded axially. In this case, the plate should be applied on the side of the bone where the most severe comminution has occurred. If bone-to-bone contact can be maintained on the side of the bone opposite the plate, motion at the fracture site can be avoided by plate pre-bending, which will be discussed in detail later. When comminution of the bone on the side opposite the plate

occurs, cyclic bending will result in a significant chance of plate failure via fatigue. If a crack is present or a chip is missing on the side opposite the plate, particular efforts must be made to prevent cyclic bending of the plate. Special precautions to avoid this situation may include one or all of the following: 1) A bone graft can be applied to the gap to form a bridging callus after vascularization of the graft occurs, normally within 2–3 weeks. 2) External support, such as a cast or a brace, may be used to provide a protection from weight bearing at least in the area of the fracture. 3) A buttress plate may be applied across the gap to prevent motion at the fracture site (one of the few times the plate would be placed in compression). This plate may be satisfactorily employed in the horse only in combination with another plate and can be used in the third metacarpus where one plate is placed medially and another laterally.

Pre-bending of the plate can result in a significant decrease in motion at the fracture site. It can be used only if contact of the cortex can be achieved on the cortex opposite the plate (*trans* cortex). When a straight plate is placed on a straight bone and the bone compressed by applying tension on the plate, an asymmetric load exists on the fracture surface with large compressive forces being exerted directly beneath the plate. If, after contouring the plate to the bone, a small kink is placed in the plate over the area of the fracture so that the plate is about 1–2 mm above the bone (Fig. 2.16a), then application of the plate to the bone will cause elastic straightening of the kink in the plate with resultant compression on the cortex opposite the plate (Fig. 2.16b). Placement of all the other screws adds to the straightening of the plate and provides a more uniform compression across the fracture site (Fig. 2.16c). In this way, small bending loads, which might tend to open the fracture site, can be avoided. This is particularly important when dealing with a bone that is axially loaded and does not appear to have a tension surface, e.g., the third metacarpus.

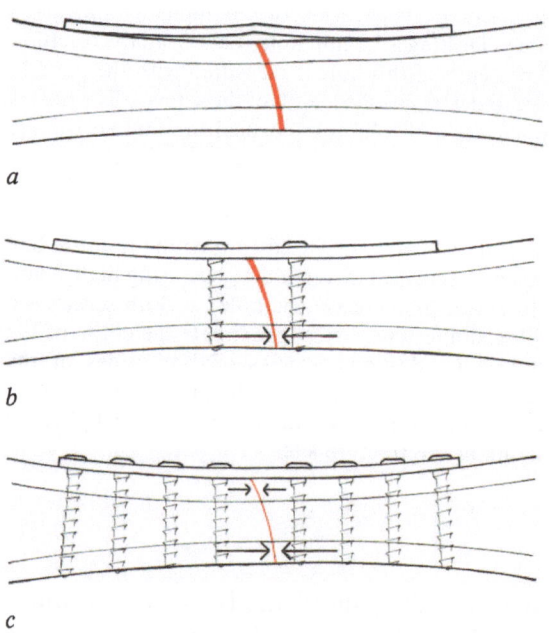

Fig. 2.16a–c. *a* The pre-bent plate is placed over the fracture with 2 mm of overbending. *b* Insertion of the initial screws causes the plate to straighten elastically, providing compression at the *trans* cortex. *c* Placement of all the other screws adds to the straightening of the plate and provides a more uniform compression across the fracture site.

When using the DCP, additional stability can be achieved by adding an interfragmentary screw through the plate and across the fracture line. The combination of pre-bending of the plate and the application of a lag screw through the plate and across the fracture line will give the best stability when using a plate for internal fixation (Fig. 2.17). This technique may only be used when there is no defect on the side opposite the plate. If a defect is present, pre-bending would change the long axis of the bone resulting in a deformity.

A plate is held against the bone by multiple screws. The purpose of the screw is to compress the plate against the bone, increasing the friction between the bone and the plate, thus preventing relative motion between them. This compressive force exerted by the screw along its axis is used to provide the bone-plate friction, which can be up to 37% of the axial force generated by the screw. Therefore, the greater the number of screws used, the more bone-plate friction is generated and the higher the weight-bearing load that can be withstood before shifting occurs between bone and plate.

The strength of a screw is in tension or compression only. The screw's function is to provide bone-plate friction, which is accomplished when the screw is under tension loading. If misused, the screw can be subjected to bending or shearing forces that will cause it to break, resulting in collapse of the internal fixation.

To obtain high bone-plate frictional forces and to protect the screws from bending or shearing loads, the plate must be contoured exactly to the surface of the bone on which it is applied. This contouring is done at the time of surgery, using bending pliers or a bending press. It is important to bend the plate adequately but only where needed since repetitive bending of the plate back and forth decreases ductility, making the steel more brittle, and predisposes to failure. Gentle bending in one direction only will work-harden the material and actually may increase its strength slightly. For perfect

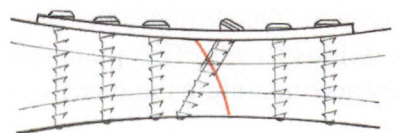

Fig. 2.17. To achieve optimal stability, pre-bending of the plate can be combined with lag screw fixation through the plate.

contouring, a slight twist of the plate may be necessary. This may be best accomplished with the bending irons. When the plate is perfectly contoured to the bone, the screws can exert their axial compression to provide a uniform distribution of the bone–plate friction which, as mentioned, is necessary to maintain the integrity of the repaired fracture.

The use of axial compression with a plate is helpful only when there are two ends of a transversely fractured bone that should be in contact. In most cases of long-bone fractures in the horse, the fracture is not transverse, and there may be many fragments with no chance for the main fragments to be compressed together axially. Therefore, other means of stabilization must be used. In these cases, interfragmentary compression, obtained with the use of lag screws, is the answer. Lag screws can be used in conjunction with the plate, as previously described under simple screw fixation, or they may be applied through the plate in order to provide the needed interfragmentary compression. Whenever possible, they should be used in combination with plate fixation. The use of lag screws represents one of the most important concepts in plate fixation when dealing with long-bone fractures in the horse. In a badly comminuted fracture, the larger fragments may be fixed to the shaft by this method. Occasionally, after several such fragments have been replaced with lag screws, the fractured ends can be reduced and stabilized with a plate. The DCP will permit a considerable amount of angulation of the screw in the slotted hole, preventing any deleterious efable amount of angulation of the screw in the slotted hole, preventing any deleterious effects. This plate therefore, can easily accommodate the interfragmentary lag screw.

Any fracture in the horse that contains the slightest defect or crack when reduced and stabilized with a plate and screws, is in need of a cancellous bone graft. Such a bone graft should be applied to fill the defect or crack as well as to extend beyond it. The resulting revascularization with calcification of the graft will form a strong and adequate callus to prevent failure of the internal fixation. Overzealous use of a cancellous bone graft will probably never pose a problem.

2.3 Cerclage

Cerclage fixation by means of wiring, is a little-used technique for internal fixation in the horse. It can be employed as a temporary fixation method prior to definitive stabilization with a plate and screws. Occasionally, cerclage wire may be helpful as a tension band wire to stabilize bony avulsion injuries and in jaw fractures. The technique of tension band wiring can be used in combination with screws to modify growth rates in the open physes of long bones (see Ch. 6).

References

Aeberhard, HJ: Der Einfluß der Platten über Biegung auf die Torsionsstabilität der Osteosynthese. Thesis, Bern Switzerland, 1973

Askew, MJ, Mow, VC: Analysis of the intraosseous stress field due to compression plating. J. Biomech. *8* (1975): 203

Hayes, WC, Perren, SM: Plate-bone friction in the compression fixation of fractures. Clinical Orthop. *89* (1972): 236

Hayes, WC, Grens WB, Murch, SA, Nunamaker, DM: Effects of plate modulus, thickness and prebending on the mechanics of compression plate fixation. Transactions of the 24th Annual Orthopaedic Research Society, 1978

Matthews, LS, Hirsch, C: Temperatures measured in human cortical bone when drilling. J. B. J. S. *54A* (1972): 297

Nunamaker, DM, Perren, SM: Force measurements in screw fixation. J. Biomech. *9* (1976): 669

Nunamaker, DM, Perren, SM: A radiological and histological analysis of fracture healing using prebending of compression plates. Clinical Orthop. *138* (1979): 167

Rybicki, EF, Simonen, F, Mills, EJ, et al: Mathematical and experimental studies on the mechanics of plated transverse fractures. J. Biomech. *7* (1974): 377

Chapter 3. Preoperative, Operative, and Postoperative Considerations

3.1 Preoperative Considerations

The following is intended as a guide for the preparation of the horse for an elective orthopedic procedure. As we have gained more experience with the management of seriously injured horses, more cases have moved out of the emergency category into a more elective mode. We feel that this has improved our results by allowing time for planning and the assemblage of appropriate staff.

3.1.1 Protection and Transport of the Injured Patient

At the time of injury the animal must be protected from further, self-inflicted injury. Horses in severe pain may seek to rid themselves of that pain by running, kicking, rolling, or a variety of other maneuvers, none of which is conducive to improving the situation. Horses with milder injuries (most carpal fractures, some fractures of the metacarpus and phalanges) may be surprisingly comfortable soon after an injury and bring danger upon themselves by appearing sound enough to continue work. A careful examination will usually reveal the pathology present, even if not in the peracute stage, and allow treatment before the situation deteriorates.

Pain should be alleviated by the judicious use of analgesics such as morphine derivatives or phenylbutazone. Anxiety might be relieved by the administration of ataractic agents. In any given case, the animal should be only brought to that point where it is no longer liable to destroy what remains of its injured extremity. Rendering the animal completely unaware of its plight by the use of heavy sedation or even general anesthesia appears contraindicated. Due consideration must also be given to the patient's general condition with regard to shock, hemorrhage, and state of hydration before deciding upon which drugs to administer. Most sedatives and tranquilizers can have profound effects on the circulatory system, and a thorough familiarity with the pharmacodynamics of those agents is essential to their successful employment in an emergency.

For an unstable fracture, especially of the limb proximal to the fetlock and distal to the elbow or stifle, the bulky bandage (Robert Jones dressing) reinforced with wooden splints or metal bars, appears to be most acceptable. All veterinarians dealing with horses to any extent might well be called upon to attend emergency fracture cases, and they should have at their disposal in ready-to-use kit form all that is necessary to meaningfully stabilize a seriously injured extremity. In the case of the Robert Jones dressing, this would mean approximately 10 pounds of cotton, 6 rolls of gauze bandage, 12 rolls of elastic bandage, and appropriate hardwood or metal splintage. The cotton is applied to the limb, producing a large, bulky cylindrical shape filling in all contours of the limb. Gauze is used to tighten the bandage provisionally, the strong elastic material is used to produce the final solid restraining dressing. When complete, the dressing should feel hard and produce a sound like a ripe melon when tapped. Splintage is applied to the outer surface of the dressing. Here, elastic or elastic adhesive bandage is employed to fix the splints in position medially, laterally, anteriorly, and posteriorly. Sufficient pressure is applied to cause the splints to indent the surface of the dressing and care is taken not to allow the tops of the splints to protrude far enough to cause soft-tissue injury (especially true of the medial splint).

When, for whatever reason, the person attending the animal does not have access to all of the above materials, a respectable fixation can be achieved by the use of pillows in place of cotton; twine or leg-wraps as bandage material; and the handles of implements such as twitches, shovels, rakes, or pitchforks as splints.

Wounds should be covered with a nonsticking dressing, and unless hemorrhage appears life-threatening, it should not be explored until appropriate preparations have been made. Especially where surgical repair is anticipated, appropriate antibiotic cover should be initiated and should include tetanus prophylaxis.

Casts might be applied to injuries of the more distal extremity and are especially useful in protecting a minimally displaced fracture during a long journey. They do, however, require specific materials and somewhat more experience in their application.

The animal with external fixation in place, especially of the more extensive types, should be assisted by at least two persons whenever moved. As transportation is planned, due consideration should be given to the smoothness of the ride (van vs trailer); ease of ingress at the farm or site of the accident; and, ease of egress at the ultimate destination (steepness of ramps, availability of loading docks). Bales of hay or straw placed around and under the animal are often helpful in stabilizing it during transport. Horses with severe injuries will often "sit" on bales placed behind them at about the height of their hamstrings to relieve the load on their extremities.

The animal might be placed in the transport vehicle facing backwards so as to protect it against unexpected jolts during an abrupt stop. Putting the vehicle back in motion is a maneuver completely under the driver's control and should be done smoothly so as never to jolt the animal.

3.1.2 Preparation of the Patient for Surgery

Owners and trainers of injured animals (especially racehorses) should be carefully questioned as to any medication that was administered to the horse prior to injury. Of particular interest is whether corticosteroids have been employed either systemically or intra-articularly. Whether organophosphate anthelmintics have been recently given might also have bearing on the patient's intraoperative management.

Any drug sensitivities should be duly recorded. Adverse reactions to specific tranquilizers, sedatives, or anesthetics should be explored.

Recent illness, such as upper respiratory infection or colic, should become part of the history, as should the animal's routine feeding program. Postoperative anorexia might have nothing to do with the primary lesion but be referable to secondary problems or management practices.

A complete physical examination and blood profile are performed. If practicable, shoes are removed and the operative site is clipped and scrubbed. Legs are prepared circumferentially from the coronary band to at least eight inches proximal to the incision site. Any additional radiographs necessary should be obtained and the limb bandaged in a sterile wrap. Feed is withheld for 12 hours preoperatively; and if prophylactic antibiotics are to be used, the administration of these drugs is instituted at this time. Our routine is to begin the administration of

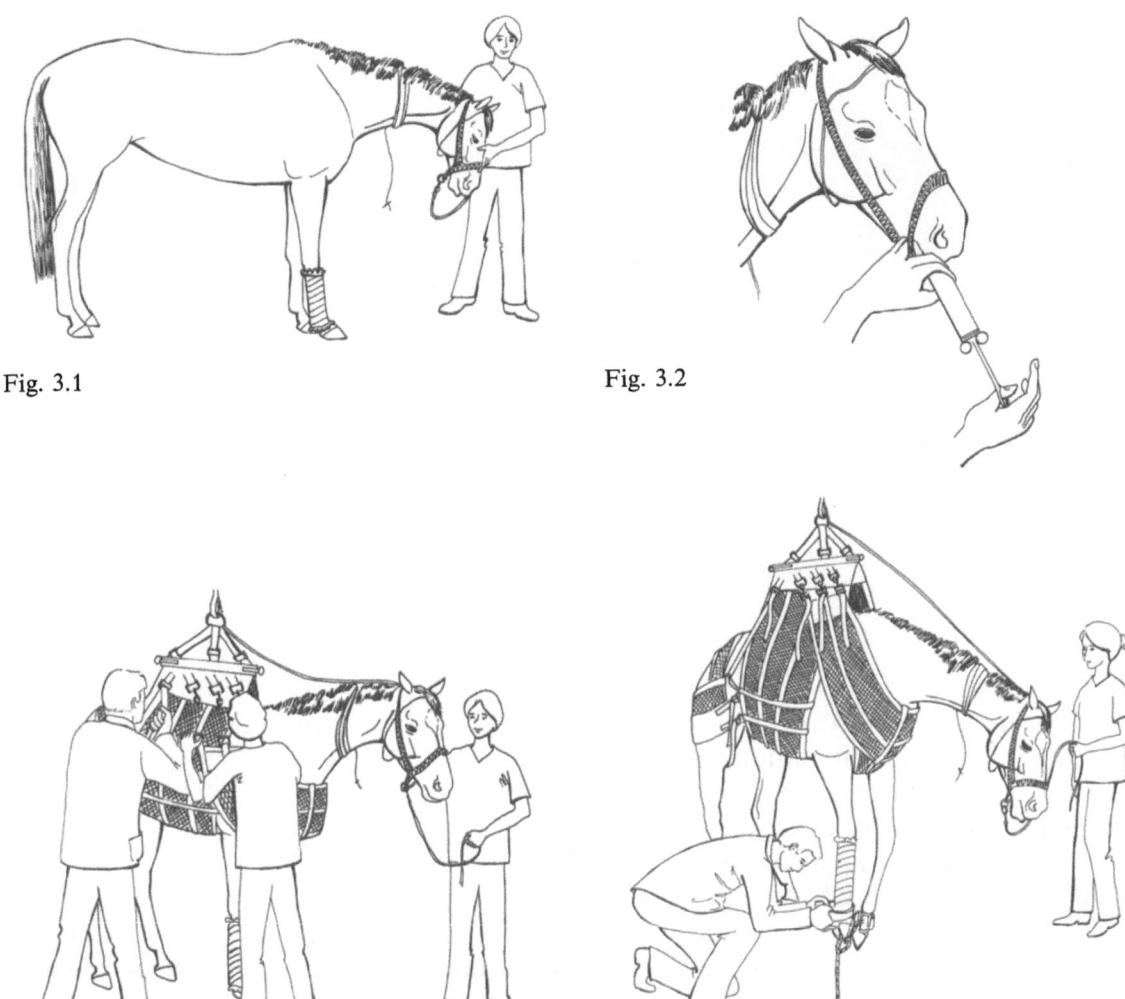

Fig. 3.1

Fig. 3.2

Fig. 3.3

Fig. 3.4

antibiotics 12 hours preoperatively and to administer them on the day of surgery and the day following surgery. This schedule might be altered in cases of contamination or severe soft-tissue trauma.

3.1.3 Anesthesia

The horse is sedated and a jugular catheter is inserted in the side of the neck that will be uppermost during surgery. Human contact is maintained during this time to keep the animal calm (Fig. 3.1). The feet are cleansed and washed, and any protective bandaging made necessary by subsequent restraint is applied. The mouth is rinsed free of any debris preparatory to endotracheal intubation (Fig. 3.2).

A nylon-polyester sling is applied and attached to an overhead monorail-hoist system (Fig. 3.3). Anesthesia is induced with a barbiturate-muscle relaxant combination, and the animal slumps into the sling. Hobbles are applied to the pasterns to aid in restraint and provide for ease of positioning the patient at a later stage (Fig. 3.4).

The horse is drawn along the monorail to the surgical theater and positioned on a

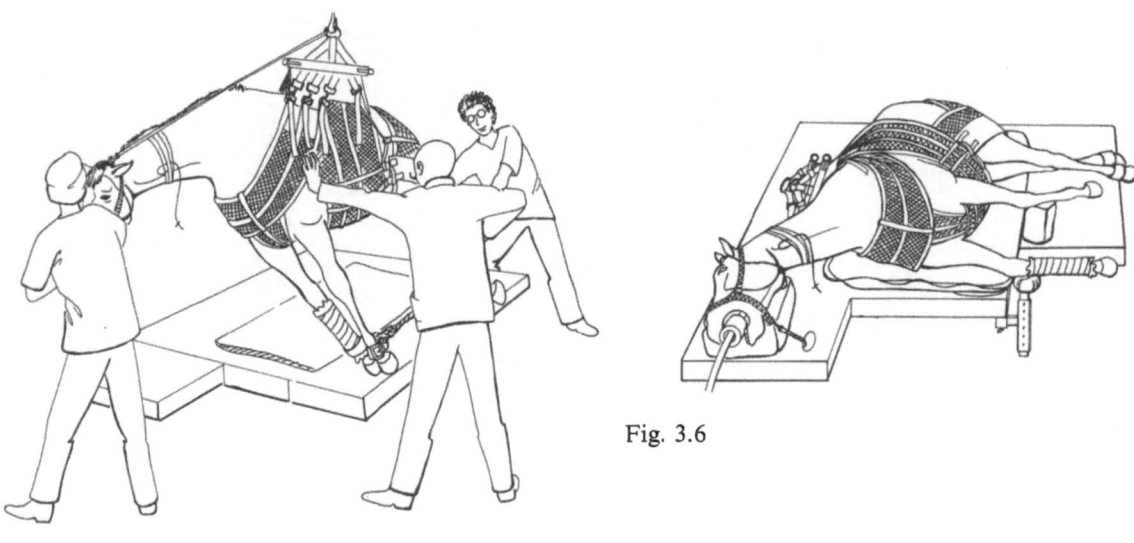

Fig. 3.5

Fig. 3.6

deflated air-mattress on the operating table (Fig. 3.5). Endotracheal intubation is carried out, the air-mattress is inflated just enough to lift the animal from the table surface, and the limbs are positioned appropriately to the particular operative procedure. The sling is loosened but allowed to remain in place to transport the horse later to the recovery facility (Fig. 3.6). Anesthesia is maintained by a mixture of a volatile agent and oxygen. Pulse, respiration, electrocardiogram, and blood pressure are monitored. The degree of peripheral perfusion is checked periodically, as are ocular and anal reflexes. Monitoring rectal and body surface temperatures can be helpful in early detection of the development of a malignant-hyperthermia-like syndrome.

3.1.4 Positioning of the Patient

When positioning the patient consideration is given to: adequate padding especially of bony prominences and large muscle masses; the surgeon's access to the operative site; the convenience and efficiency with which drapes can be applied; and, the ability to perform intraoperative radiographic examinations without breaking asepsis.

3.2 Operative Considerations

3.2.1 Aseptic Technique

The operating room is closed off from other areas, and any special airflow or filtering systems are activated. Any personnel to remain with the horse during surgery don appropriate clothing, caps, masks, and shoe covers. The surgeon, or surgeons, retire to the scrub facility.

Rubber gloves or other protective devices are applied to the patient's hooves, and the entire body, save the limb upon which surgery will be performed, is covered with non-sterile red cloth shrouds. The wraps placed on the extremity the previous day are then removed.

If an Esmarch's bandage or tourniquet is to be used, it is applied at this juncture. Many surgeons opt to apply this local exsanguination at a later stage, while some (including the authors) dispense with it altogether.

The limb is finally prepared for aseptic surgery circumferentially for at least eight inches proximal and distal to the surgical

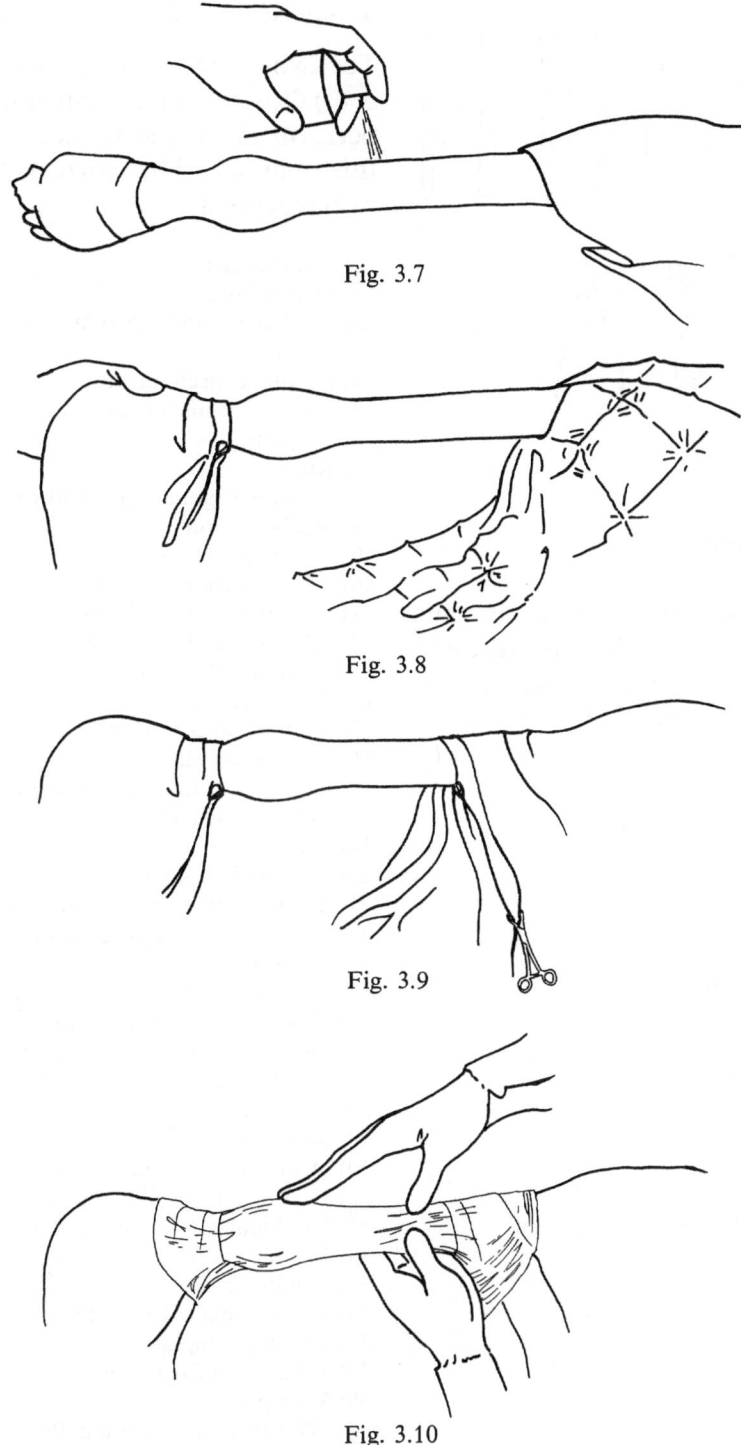

Fig. 3.7

Fig. 3.8

Fig. 3.9

Fig. 3.10

site. Following scrubbing and disinfection, the limb is dried, and a spray adhesive is applied (Fig. 3.7).

A sterile impervious plastic split sheet is positioned beneath the limb and encircling it above the operative site (Fig. 3.8). Sterile cloth shrouds are placed encircling the limb above and below the operative site (Fig. 3.9).

Adhesive transparent draping material is applied to the operative site and smoothed into position especially along the intended line of incision (Fig. 3.10).

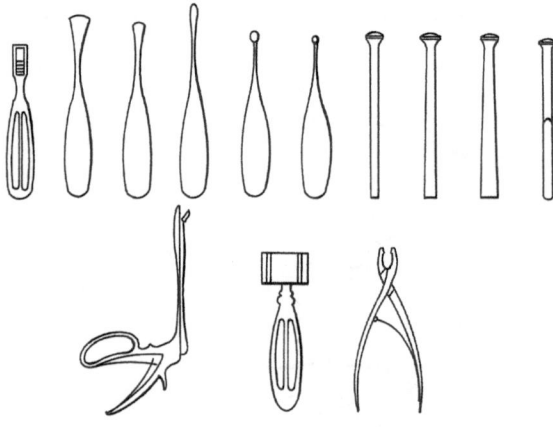

Fig. 3.11

3.2.2 Instrumentation

In addition to the assortment of instruments listed below, which are used for exposure and soft-tissue dissection, the illustrated set of bone instruments are useful (Fig. 3.11).

a) standard soft-tissue set
Scapel(s)
1 pair Mayo scissors (curved blunt)
1 pair Metzenbaum scissors (curved blunt)
Thumb forceps

6 Allis tissue forceps
8 Kelly hemostatic forceps
8 Mosquito hemostatic forceps
12 Backhaus towel clamps
1 Mayo Hegar needle holder
1 Foerster sponge forceps (curved)

Volkmann retractors (4 prong blunt and sharp)
Saline basin
Bulb syringe

b) standard bone set (Fig. 3.11, left to right)
Mathieu raspatory
Langenbeck periosteal elevators
  broad sharp
  broad blunt
  narrow blunt
Bruns oval cup curettes
  size 2
  size 4
US Army-pattern osteotomes
  6 mm
  12 mm
  18 mm
US Army gouge — 10 mm
Ferris-Smith straight cup jaw rongeur — 4 × 10 mm
Crane bone mallet (225 gm)
Lane bone rongeur (large jaw) — 6 cm

Standard ASIF large animal instrumentation

The two composite diagrams (Figs. 3.12 and 3.13) illustrate those instruments required to perform all of the procedures described in this manual. The correct names for the instruments are:

1) Countersink
2) Depth gauge
3) tap handle and 4.5 mm taps (regular and extra long)
4) 6.5 mm cancellous tap
5) Standard screwdriver and screwdriver for quick coupling
6) Ruler
7) 8 mm hexagonal open-end wrench (for nuts)
8) Small air drill
9) Sesamoid clamp
10) 4.5 mm drill bit — extra long (170 mm)
11) 4.5 mm drill bit (120 mm)
12) 3.2 mm drill bit — extra long (170 mm)
13) 3.2 mm drill bit (120 mm)
14) 2 mm drill bit
15) 6.5 mm cancellous tap sleeve
16) 3.5 mm tap sleeve
17) 4.5 mm tap sleeve and plate protector
18) Equine C-clamp
19) C-clamp
20) 3.2 mm drill sleeve
21) 22 mm wide-tipped Hohmann retractor
22) 18 mm narrow-tipped Hohmann retractor
23) Sharp hook
24) 35 mm wide-tipped Hohmann retractor
25) 43 mm narrow-tipped Hohmann retractor
26) Drill sleeve for tension device
27) Tension device — span 16 mm
28) Pin wrench
29) Socket wrench
30) Open-end and box wrench — 11 mm
31) DCP neutral drill guide, *green*
32) DCP load drill guide, *yellow*
33) Bending iron
34) Bending press
35) Bending pliers for plates
36) Bending templates
37) 1.2 mm cerclage wire
38) Wire passer
39) Wire tightener with handle
40) Wire cutters
41) Speed-lock reduction forceps — 220 mm
42) Self-centering bone-holding forceps — size 3

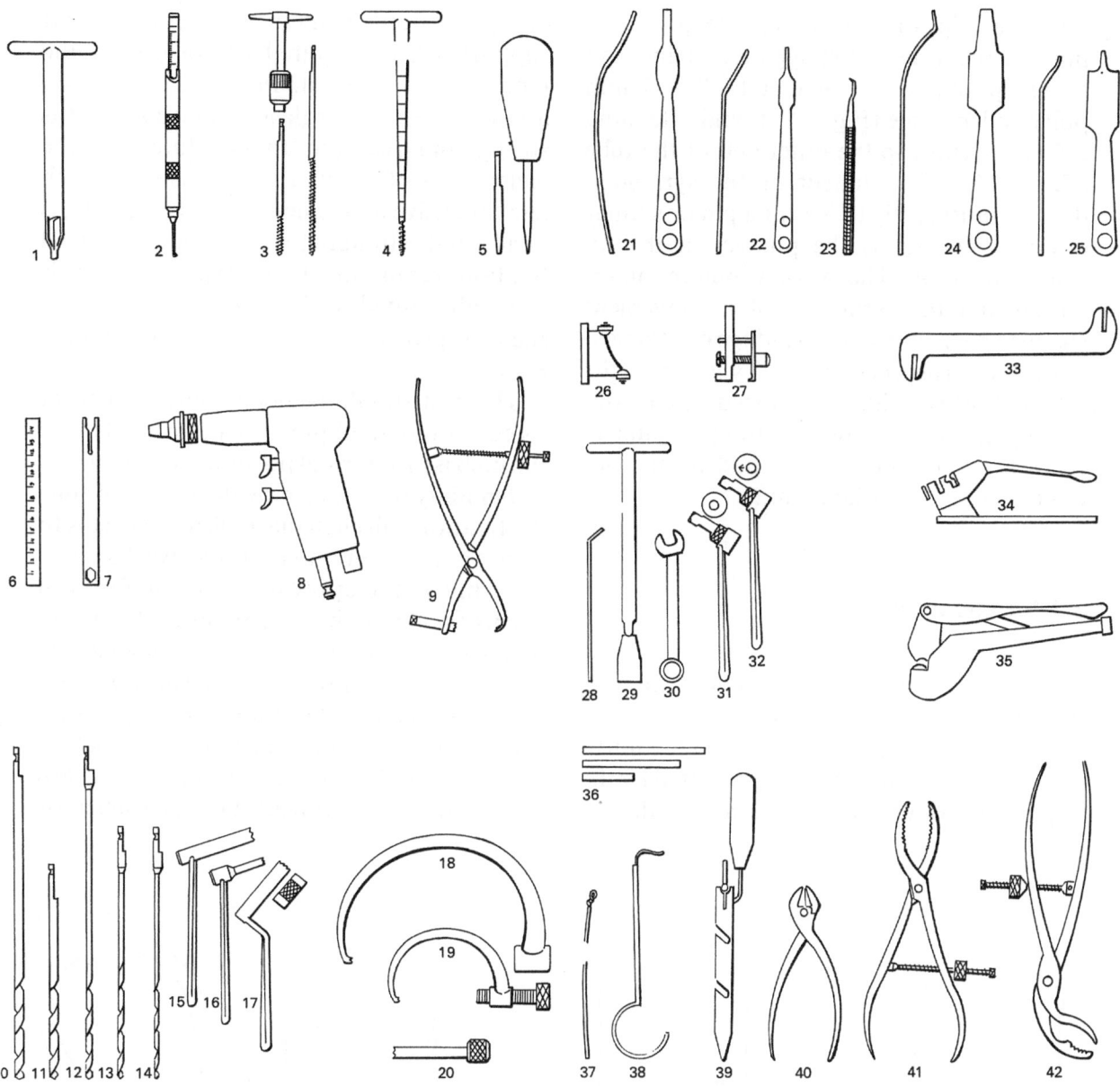

Fig. 3.12 (Not to scale.)　　　　Fig. 3.13 (Not to scale.)

3.3 Postoperative Considerations

3.3.1 Drainage

Postoperative drainage is especially important in areas of extensive soft-tissue damage or wide exposure. Exudate and/or blood must be eliminated from the surgical site if good soft-tissue healing without infection is

to occur. Of the many forms of drainage available, the suction drainage system seems superior since it is more effective in removing fluid from the surgical site, may be removed independent of external fixation devices, and provides an ingress pathway for the local administration of antibiotics.

Installation of a suction drainage system may be accomplished by: tunneling under the skin proximal to the surgical site with hemostatic forceps; making a stab incision over the tip of the forceps (Fig. 3.14); pushing the forceps through the stab incision to grasp the fenestrated end of a 5 mm polyethylene tube (Fig. 3.15); and attaching a 50 ml syringe to the outer end of the tube (Fig. 3.16). The plunger of the syringe is drilled transversely to accept a pin or similar device which holds the plunger in the retracted position. The suction thus created is strong and the syringe is of a convenient shape to be included in a bandage or attached to the lateral aspect of a cast. Twice daily, the tube is flushed with heparinized saline containing antibiotics, and the drain remains in place until the amount of fluid being conducted becomes insignificant.

3.3.2 External Fixation

When the internal fixation devices applied cannot be relied upon to confer stability under weight-bearing conditions, they must, as discussed in Chapter 2, be protected by the application of external fixation. The degree of support needed and the length of time that support will be required will determine the type of fixation used. For longer-term fixation, we use a fiberglass bandage since it is strong and resistant to moisture and the vicissitudes of life in a stall. Plaster is much less expensive and, when applied correctly, is of adequate strength for many or all external fixation requirements in the horse. It is especially suited to short-term applications, such as protection of the limb during the recovery phase.

The cast should be adequately padded at its edges and at all pressure points. Whether the limb is in a normal position or extended is also mainly determined by the length of time the fixation will be in place. When a cast is to stay on for more than three weeks, it is probably best to apply it with the limb in full extension. Though this creates a "long leg" on the operated side, this can be alleviated by building up the opposite foot. This positioning prevents the development of pressure sores at the posterior aspect of the fetlock or breakage of the cast in the fetlock-pastern area. Some protection, be it metal, rubber, or

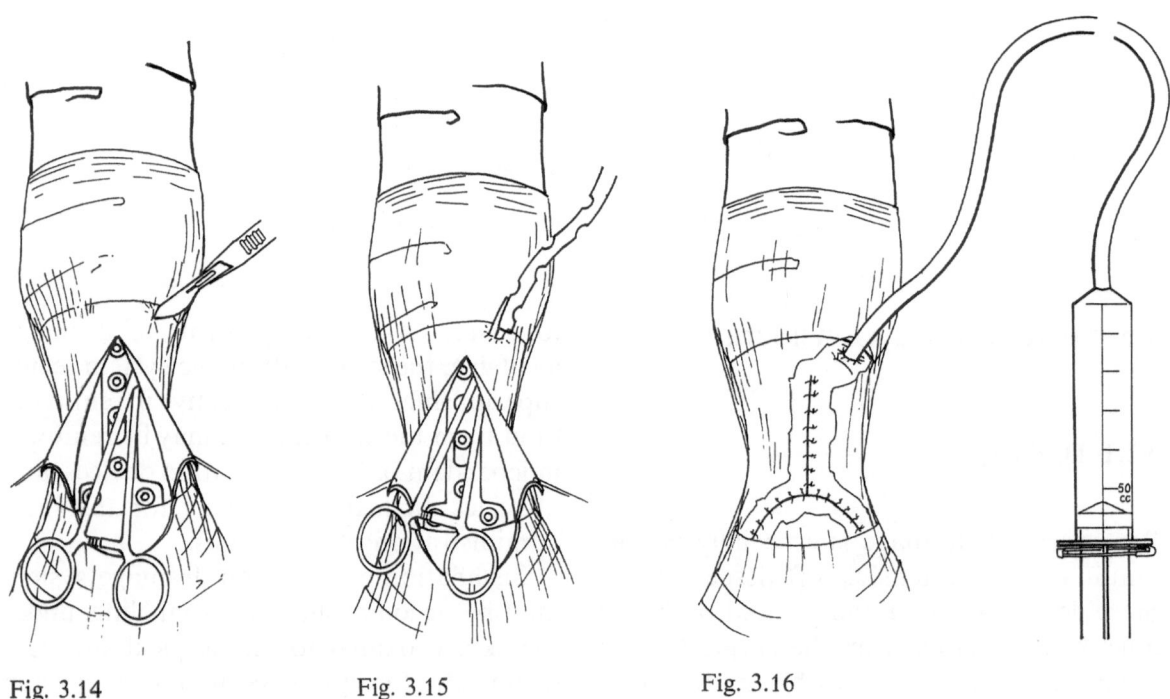

Fig. 3.14   Fig. 3.15   Fig. 3.16

other material, should be given to the bottom of the cast to prevent the foot from wearing through the cast. If this occurs, the movement of the leg relative to the cast increases markedly, and the danger of the development of abrasions increases proportionally.

When it is anticipated that the animal will be putting most of its weight upon the limb opposite to the operated extremity, the foot of that "support leg" should be packed with hard acrylic plastic. This will help to prevent the laminitis that can develop due to overload and minimize the subsequent ventral rotation of the third phalanx relative to the hoof wall.

3.3.3 Medication

When prophylactic antibiotics are used, their administration should begin prior to surgery and be continued through the day of surgery and for at least 24 hours following surgery. The type of coverage will be determined by safety, the individual surgeon's preferences and the anticipated degree and type of contamination. Where extensive soft-tissue damage is a feature of the injury, coverage should be broader and longer. When dealing with obvious infection, antibiotic' treatment is no longer truly prophylactic, and its character should be guided by the results of culture and sensitivity testing.

Analgesics should be used to improve the animal's demeanor during the phase of recovery from anesthesia and to prevent undue suffering in the convalescent period. Morphine or meperidine are potent short-term analgesics to be used early during recovery, while phenylbutazone is a dependable drug to be used later over a more protracted period. Except for some extremely high doses or very long treatment periods, the drug appears to be without deleterious side effects in the horse.

3.3.4 Exercise

Individual postoperative exercise schedules are discussed in later chapters on specific injuries and assume access to the usual facilities at a farm or training center. In general, we attempt to begin moving an extremity as soon as possible following surgery without endangering fixation devices or the structure repaired. This may mean restriction to a stall and only passive manipulation of the limb in more serious injuries or very soon following surgery. In more stable situations, handwalking might be instituted at one week postoperatively.

If facilities permit, swimming exercise can be employed to great advantage as soon as soft-tissue healing is complete (2–3 weeks postoperatively and throughout the convalescent period). Edematous swelling of the operated limb is reduced, range of motion of any associated joint is improved, and the animal's general condition is maintained. Allowing a horse to become as physically unfit as the usual "turnout" situation permits most certainly predisposes it to renewed injury when training or competition is resumed. While swimming cannot condition a horse totally for racing competition, it can sustain the capabilities of the cardiopulmonary systems and significantly help to maintain fitness of the musculoskeletal system.

References

Altemeier, WA, Hummel, RP, Hull, EO, and Lewis, BA: Changing patterns in surgical infections. Ann. Surg. *178* (1973): 436-445

Bowmann, KF, Fackelman, GE: Comminuted fractures in the horse. Comp. Vet. Educ. *2* (1980): 98-102

Rittmann, WW, Sehibli, M, Matter, P, and Allgöwer, M: Open fractures—long term results in 200 consecutive cases. Clin Orthop. *138* (1979): 132-140

Thomas, DP, Fregin, GF Gerber, NH, and Ailes, NB: Cardiorespiratory adjustments to tethered swimming in the horse. Pflügers Arch. *385* (1980): 65-70

Kennedy, JC, Hawkins, R, and Krissoff, WB: Orthopaedic manifestations of swimming. Am. J. Sports Med. *6* (1978): 309-322

Waldron-Mease, E, Rosenberg, H: Post-anesthetic myositis in the horse associated with in vitro malignant hypertermia susceptibility. Vet. Sci. Commun. *3* (1979): 45-50

Part II

Part II

Chapter 4. Fractures Amenable to Treatment by Lag Screw Fixation

4.1 Carpal Fractures

The most common fracture of the carpus presented for internal fixation is the slab fracture of the anterior or anteromedial aspect of the third carpal bone.

To *approach* this region of the carpus, an incision is made close to the axial aspect of the tendon of the extensor carpi radialis. The incision is begun at the level of the middle of the radial carpal bone proximally and ends at the level of the carpometacarpal joint (Fig. 4.1) A similar incision is made into the intercarpal joint (Fig. 4.2). Synovectomy of the proliferative membranous portion of the joint capsule is frequently performed to improve access to the joint and visualization of the fracture site.

The proximal joint surface of the third carpal bone is carefully examined to determine the exact plane of the fracture and to assess any attendant cartilaginous damage (Fig. 4.3). The distal articular surface of the corresponding radial carpal bone is similarly evaluated for the presence of arthritic change

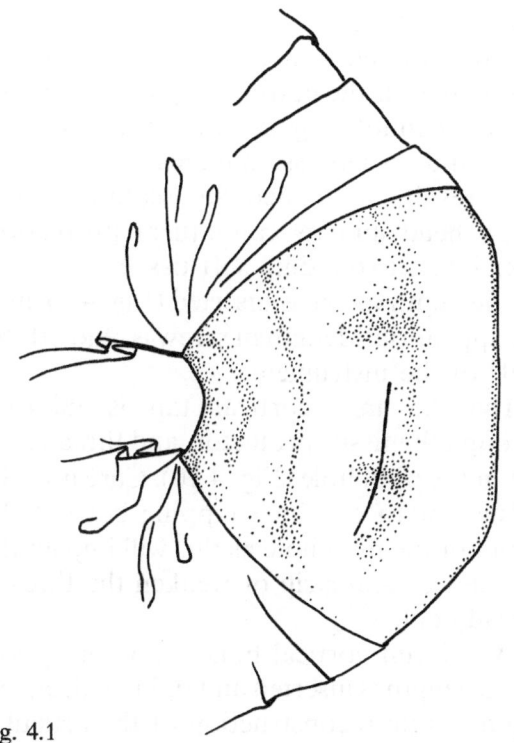

Fig. 4.1

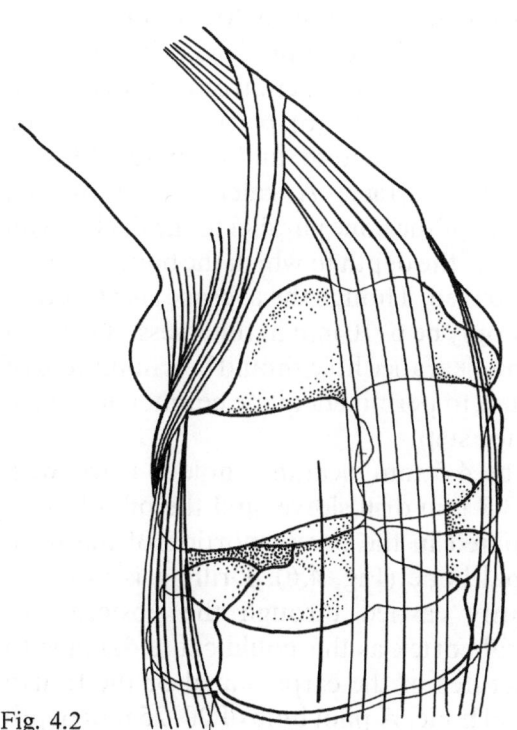

Fig. 4.2

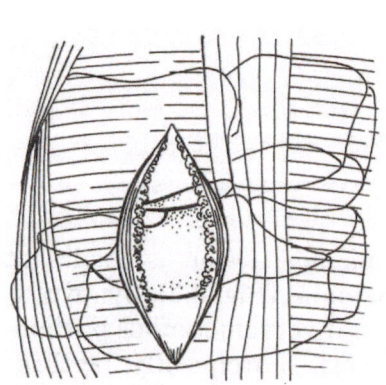

Fig. 4.3

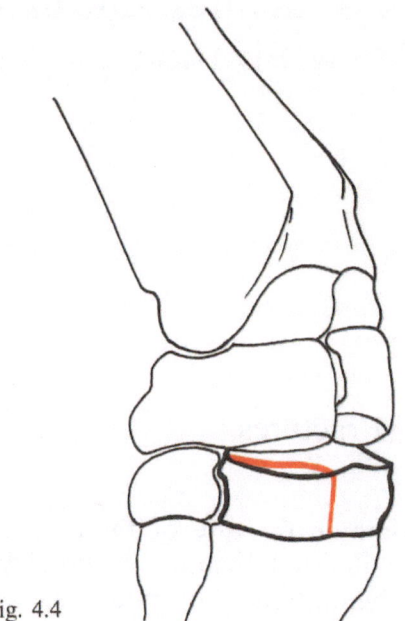

Fig. 4.4

(Fig. 4.4). Any bony fragments or cartilaginous debris are removed by direct extirpation or curettage.

The *surgical procedure* is depicted in Figure 4.5–4.11.

Figure 4.5 shows the 4.5 mm drill bit placed through the 4.5 mm tap sleeve. The instruments are applied to the face of the third carpal bone so that the drill bit is: (a) centered in the fragment from top to bottom and side to side: (b) perpendicular to the plane of the fracture, and (c) parallel to the articular surface. A ruler placed on the surface of the bone parallel to the drill bit will indicate the depth to which the bone has been penetrated. Though the average slab fracture may only be 6–10 mm in thickness, the depth of the clearance hole should be a minimum of 12 mm to permit adequate countersinking in a later step.

The 4.5 mm clearance hole is fitted with the 3.2 mm drill sleeve, and the pilot hole is prepared in the parent portion of the third carpal bone (Fig. 4.6). Drilling is not necessarily carried through the posterior or lateral cortex as this could cause damage to structures of the carpal canal or the fourth carpal bone. A pilot hole of 20–25 mm depth provides ample holding power for a 4.5 mm cortical bone screw.

Countersinking (Fig. 4.7) is carried out sufficiently to provide a good seat for the screw head around the entire circumference of the clearance hole. The distance from the tip of the countersink to the top of its cutting edge is 12 mm.

When the clearance hole is less than 12 mm in depth, the cutting edges of the countersink cannot engage the surface of the bone, and no depression is created (Fig. 4.8). This results in inadequate seating of the screw head and its consequent protrusion later into surrounding soft tissues.

The depth gauge is inserted (Fig. 4.9), and the appropriate length of screw is read off the scale of the instrument.

The 4.5 mm cortical tap is inserted through the tissue protector, and threads are cut in the pilot hole (Fig. 4.10). Care must be taken not to continue tapping beyond the depth of the pilot hole as this will impact the instrument and strip or weaken the threads already cut.

A 4.5 mm cortical bone screw of appropriate length is inserted and tightened, effecting accurate reconstruction of the articular surface and compression of the fracture plane (Fig. 4.11).

Postoperatively, a non-sticking gauze dressing is applied to the wound, and the limb is placed in a pressure bandage. This bandage is changed 24 hours, after surgery and replaced by sheet cotton and elastic bandage applied from the coronary band to midradius. This second dressing remains in place until skin suture removal at 7–10 days postoperatively. The patient receives 6 weeks stall rest and, for a further 6 weeks, only handwalking exercise. Radiographic evaluation is then carried out, and, given positive findings, the animal is allowed 12 weeks of exercise at will at pasture before the resumption of training. The radiographs reproduced in Fig. 4.12 a–d illustrate a typical case.

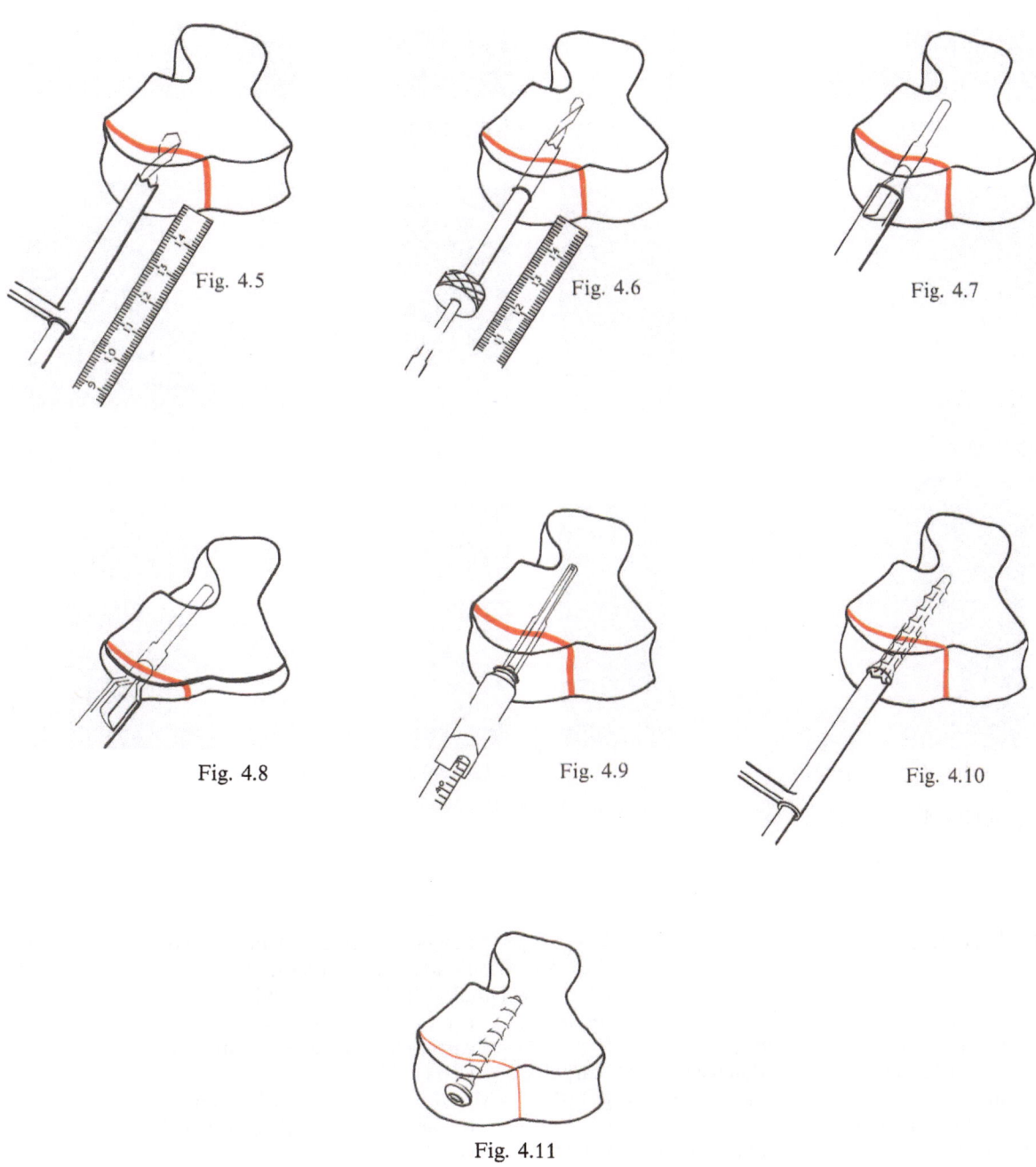

Fig. 4.5

Fig. 4.6

Fig. 4.7

Fig. 4.8

Fig. 4.9

Fig. 4.10

Fig. 4.11

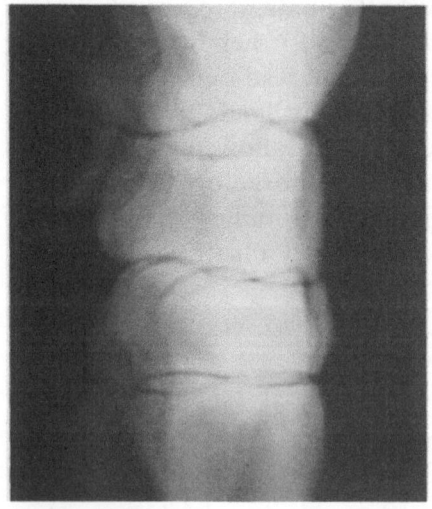

a preoperative

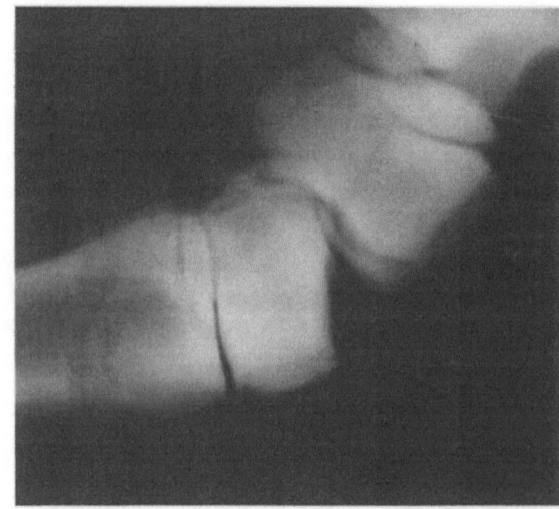

b preoperative

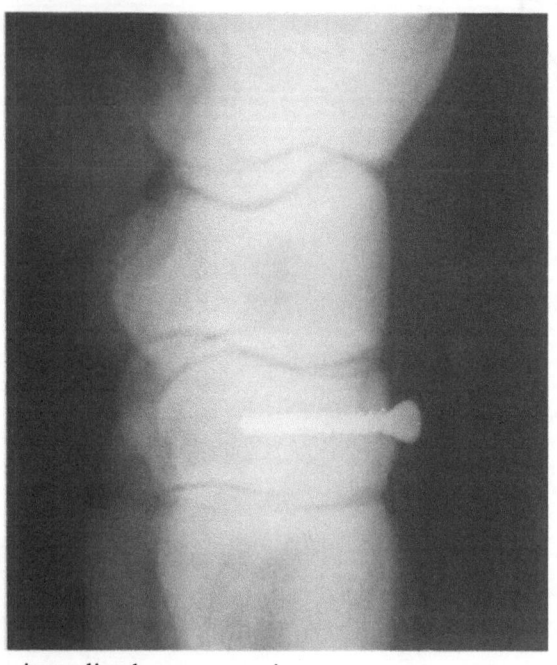

c immediately postoperative

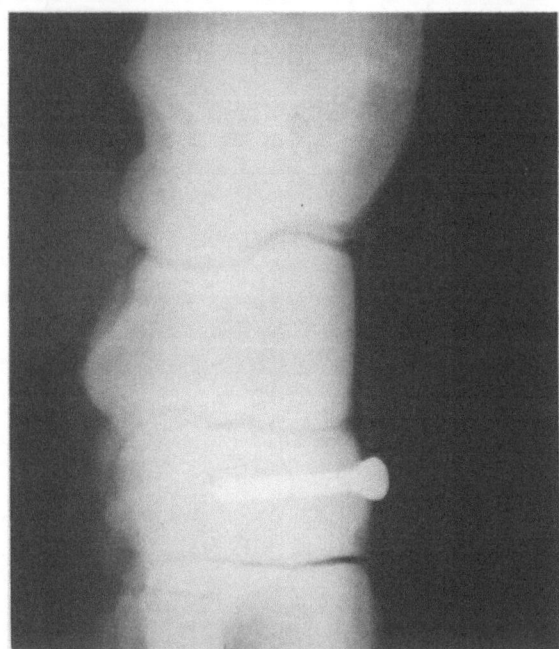

d 12 weeks postoperative

Fig. 4.12 a–d

References

Auer, J: Diseases of the carpus. *Vet. Clin. North Am.* [*Large Anim. Pract.*] *2* (1980): 81–99

Larson, LH, Dixon, RT: Management of carpal injuries in the fast gaited horse. Aust. Vet. J. *46* (1970): 133–139

Manning, JP, St. Clair, LE: Surgical repair of third carpal bone fractures in the Thoroughbred horse. Illinois Vet. *3* (1960): 106–111

Thrall, ED; Lebel, JL, and O'Brien, TR: A five year survey of the incidence and location of equine carpal chip fractures. J. Am. Vet. Med. Assoe. *158* (1971): 1366–68

Wyburn, RS, Goulden, BE: Fractures of the equine carpus: A report of 57 cases. N. Z. Vet. J. *22* (1974): 133–142

4.2 Metacarpal Fractures

4.2.1 Stress Fractures ("Saucer" or "Tongue" Fractures)

Fractures of the anterior or anterolateral cortex of the third metacarpal bone are frequently encountered in the racing Thoroughbred. There is a marked predilection for the left forelimb, and the usual age of occurrence is 3–5 years. The syndrome may be related to the microfractures and metacarpal cortical hyperplasia that occur, usually bilaterally, in younger animals, considered of less clinical significance and referred to as "bucked shins."

Some "saucer" or "tongue" fractures, as these cracks have been called due to their characteristic radiographic appearance, will heal without surgery under a program of controlled exercise alone. Others remain chronically unstable, preventing successful training, and occasionally, transverse fractures of the entire metacarpus will occur through the original unicortical defect. These facts in combination with the observation that most, if not all, of the unicortical fractures will heal faster following internal fixation have led to a general increase in the numbers of afflicted animals in which surgery seems indicated. As one considers surgery, careful preoperative evaluation of radiographs should be carried out to ascertain especially whether: (a) there are multiple fractures present in the left third metacarpal bone, or (b) there is any similar pathology present in the right third metacarpal bone.

Figure 4.13 illustrates the typical appearance of a saucer fracture as it is best visualized in the medial oblique projection of the metacarpal bone. There is characteristically some endosteal and periosteal proliferation associated with the fracture. At surgery, this proliferative bone will render the fracture line obscure, so that orientation of the implant will depend largely upon a thorough knowledge of associated anatomic structures and the exact angle at which preoperative radiographs were taken. It behooves one, therefore, to label the preoperative projections carefully.

The *surgical approach* is through a skin incision located between the common and lateral digital extensor tendons. The incision is carried through the fascia to the periosteum. A self-retaining retractor is placed parting the tendons, and the periosteum is incised and reflected. The surface of the cortex is examined for evidence of a crack or to localize the associated periosteal proliferative change precisely. Figures 4.14–4.19 describe in detail the surgical procedure.

Using preoperative radiographs to determine the appropriate angle of inclination of the drill bit in the coronal plane and anatomic landmarks (periosteal proliferative change, level of the fetlock joint, tip of the splint bone) to determine the correct proximo-distal location, the 4.5 mm drill bit is inserted through the tap sleeve and a

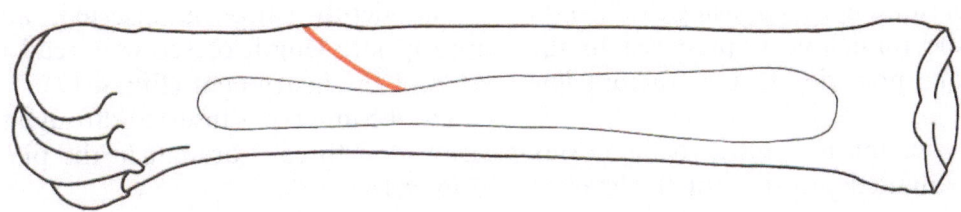

Fig. 4.13

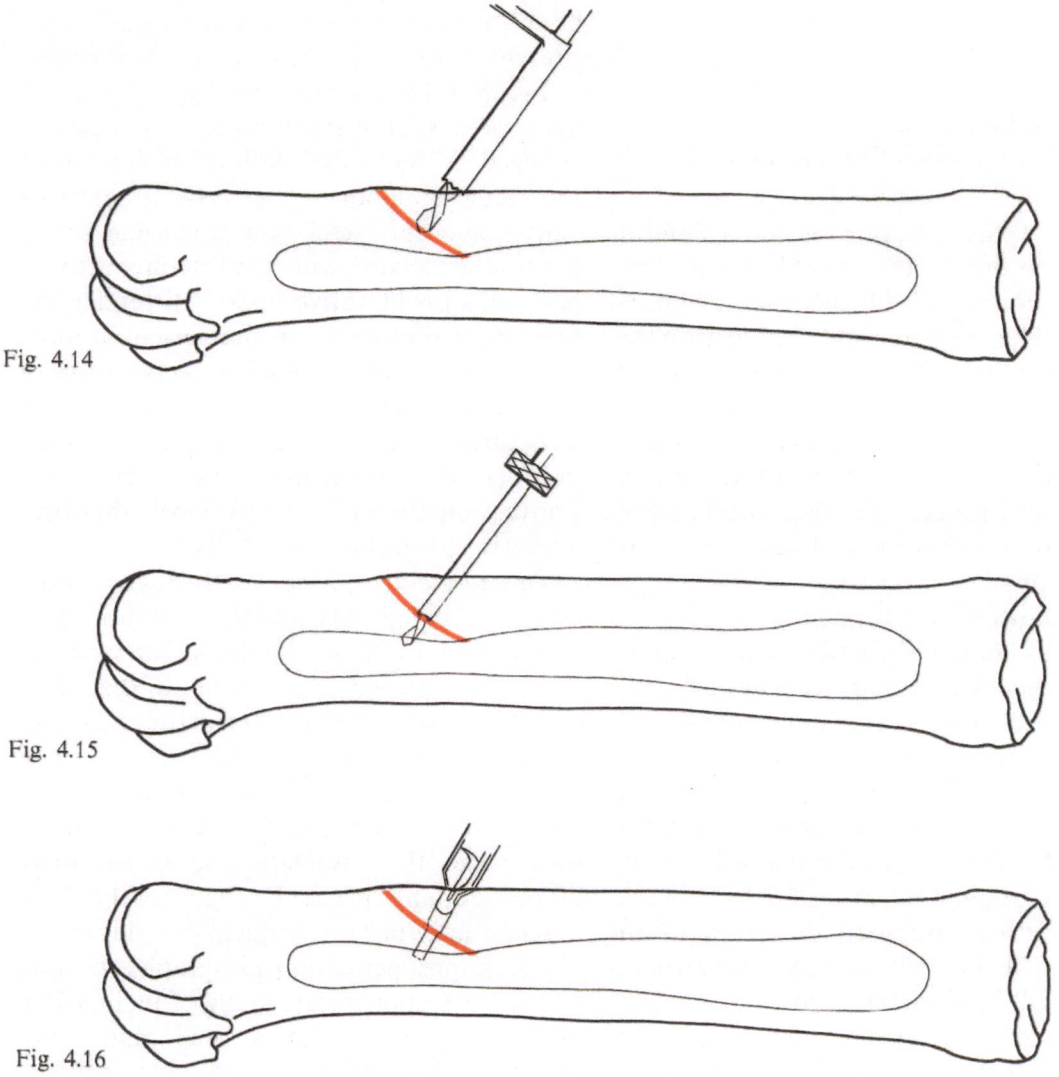

Fig. 4.14

Fig. 4.15

Fig. 4.16

clearance hole is drilled through to the fracture line (Fig. 4.14).

The clearance hole is carried to at least 12 mm in depth to allow for adequate countersinking later.

The 3.2 mm drill sleeve is inserted in the 4.5 mm clearance hole, and using the 3.2 mm drill bit, the pilot hole is prepared in the cortical bone posterior to the fracture line (Fig. 4.15).

The countersink is applied to the cortex and an adequate depression for the head of the screw is prepared (Fig. 4.16). The screw head must be well seated in the cortex to not interfere afterward with the proper function of the extensor tendons. Note that if the 4.5 mm clearance hole is not deep enough, the tip of the countersink will not penetrate the bone sufficiently to allow complete engagement of the cutting edges of the instrument.

The depth gauge is inserted, and the appropriate length of screw is read on the scale of the instrument (Fig. 4.17).

The 4.5 mm tap is inserted through the tap sleeve and threads are cut in the pilot hole (Fig. 4.18).

A cortical bone screw of appropriate length is inserted and tightened (Fig. 4.19), effecting compression of the fracture plane.

42

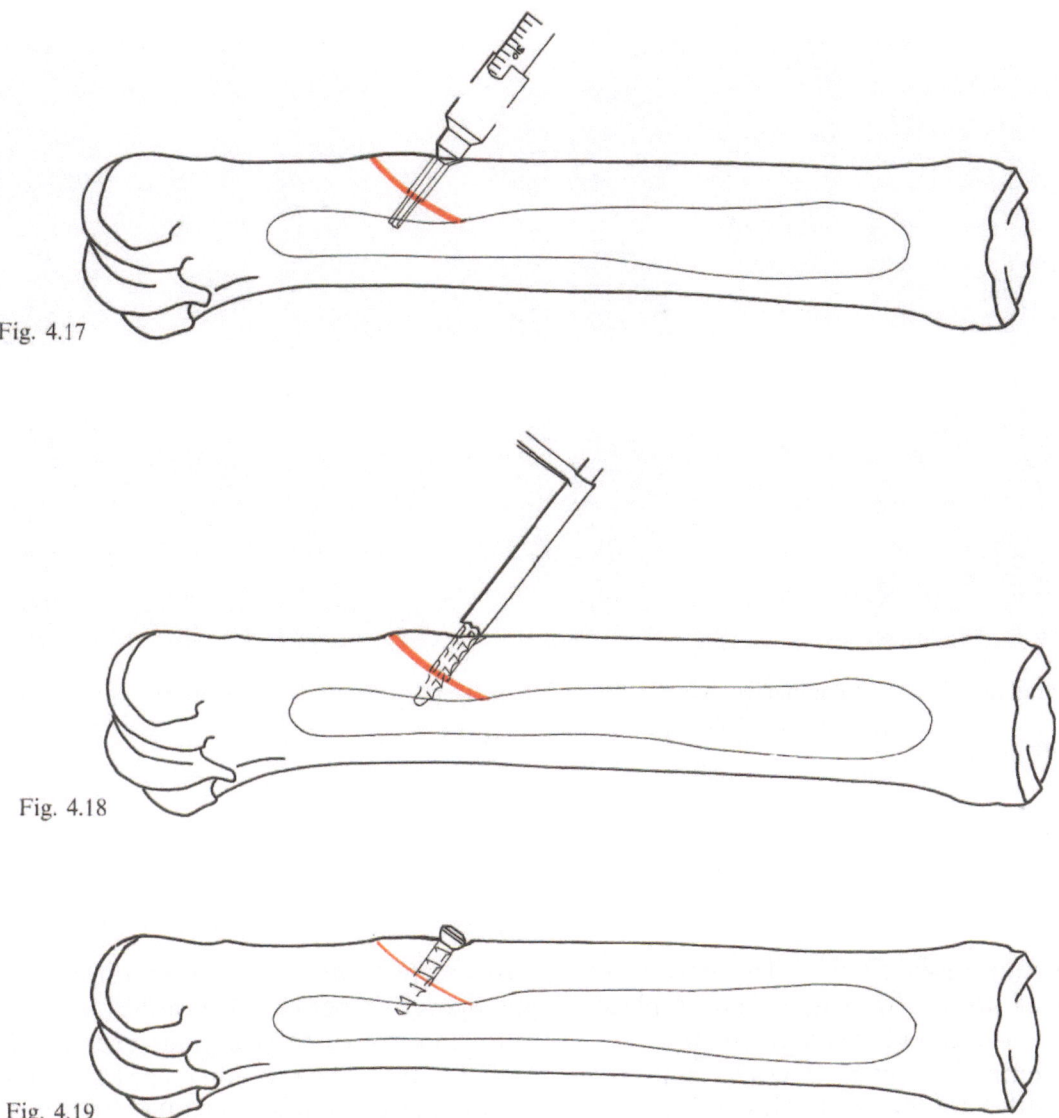

Fig. 4.17

Fig. 4.18

Fig. 4.19

Radiographs are taken on the operating table to ensure correct orientation of the implant employed.

Closure of the soft tissues is begun by placing a row of simple continuous 00 chromic catgut sutures in the periosteum and deep fascia beneath the extensor tendons drawing those layers over the screw head. The retractors are removed and the extensor tendons are permitted to return to their original position. A second row of sutures are placed in the loose areolar tissue superficial to the extensor tendons using the same material and technique, care being taken not to pierce the tendons themselves. Following the placement of several interrupted subcuticular sutures of 00 chromic catgut in horizontal mattress fashion, the skin is closed routinely.

Postoperatively, a non-sticking sterile gauze dressing is placed upon the wound, and the limb is placed in a lightly padded cast with the foot flat and the fetlock in a normal position. This cast is applied to protect the cannon bone during recovery from anesthesia, as one of the major complications of this surgery may be transverse fracture of the metacarpus through the treated or a pre-

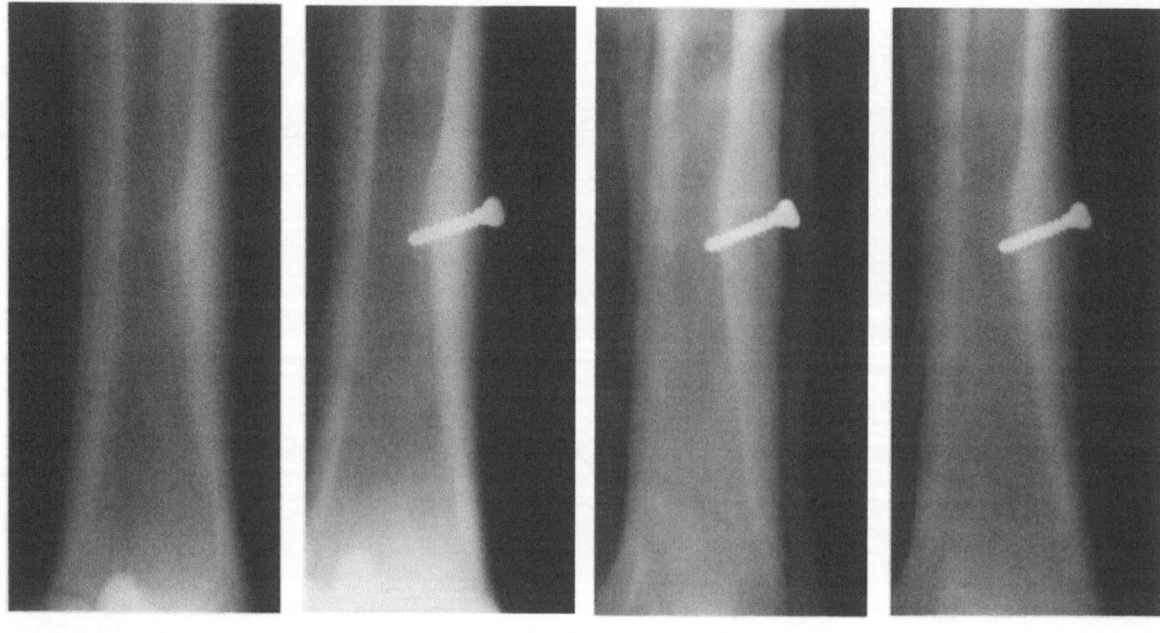

a preoperative   *b* immediately   *c* 6 weeks postoperative   *d* 12 weeks postoperative
                              postoperative

Fig. 4.20 a–d

viously unnoticed fissure. The cast is removed 24 hours after surgery and replaced by sheet cotton and elastic bandages.

The animal is given 2 weeks stall rest, followed by 4 weeks of handwalking and 6 weeks of light exercise, at first with a lead pony. At 12 weeks postoperatively, follow-up radiographs are taken, and given positive findings, the horse may be returned to fast training aimed at its first race 30 days later. The radiographs in Figure 4.20 illustrate a typical case.

Perhaps more than any other, stress or fatigue fractures of the third metacarpal bone represent a dilemma in treatment and postoperative care. The surgery can be particularly demanding as concerns spatial relations and the outcome can be quite variable dependent upon individual healing patterns and the capabilities of those observing the animal during its convalescence. In some cases operated upon, the implants them-

selves seem to have caused pain in the later postoperative period (4 months — 1 year) following return to strenuous exercise. Removal of the screws at that stage has resulted in soundness; it has also resulted in recurrence of the fracture and renewed lameness.

This technique is included here since it has been used successfully where others have failed. The problem of fatigue fractures of the third metacarpal bone remains, however, an area of active investigation, and surely a better understanding of the underlying basic pathology will lead to the development of more consistently dependable therapeutic methods.

References

Chamay, A: Mechanical and morphological aspects of experimental overload and fatigue in bone. J. Biomech. *3* (1970): 263–270

Devas, MB: Shin splints or stress fractures of the metacarpal bone in horses, and shin soreness or stress fractures of the tibia in man. J. Bone Joint Surg. *49B* (1967): 310–313

Dixon, RT, Bellenger, CR: Fissure fracture of the equine metacarpus and metatarsus. J. Am. Vet. Med. Assoc. *153* (1968): 1289–1292

Norwood, G: The bucked-shin complex. Proc. Am. Assoc. Equine Pract. *25* (1979): 88–97

Orava, S, Puranen, J, and Ala-Ketola, L: Stress fractures caused by physical exercise. Acta Orthop. Scand. *49* (1978): 19–27

Rooney, JR: Bucked shin. Mod. Vet. Pract. *56* (1978): 633–634

Wheat, JD: Bilateral fractures of the third metacarpal bone of a Thoroughbred. J. Am. Vet. Med. Assoc. *140* (1962): 815–816

4.2.2 Condylar Fractures

a) Displaced

Fractures of the distal metacarpal condyles are encountered mainly in the racing Thoroughbred, though horses competing in harness racing may also be affected. Whether the injuries occur in the left or the right forelimb, there is a marked predilection for the lateral condyle. The fractures may or may not show proximal displacement of the fragment at the joint surface (Figs. 4.21 and 4.38).

The *surgical approach* employed is dependent upon the degree of displacement. A case such as that illustrated in Figure 4.21 is approached through a double flap curvilinear incision, the distal arc of which is based anteriorly (Fig. 4.22). The periosteum, deep fascia, and distally, the joint capsule are incised along the anterior portion of the fracture line beginning at the proximal tip of the fragment and extending into the fetlock joint. The incision is carried to the level of the proximodorsal rim of the first phalanx (Figs. 4.23 and 4.24). Using an elevator, the fragment is lifted, and both sides of the fracture plane are scrupulously cleansed of bony debris or the fibrous tissue characteristic of an organizing hematoma (Fig. 4.25). Under

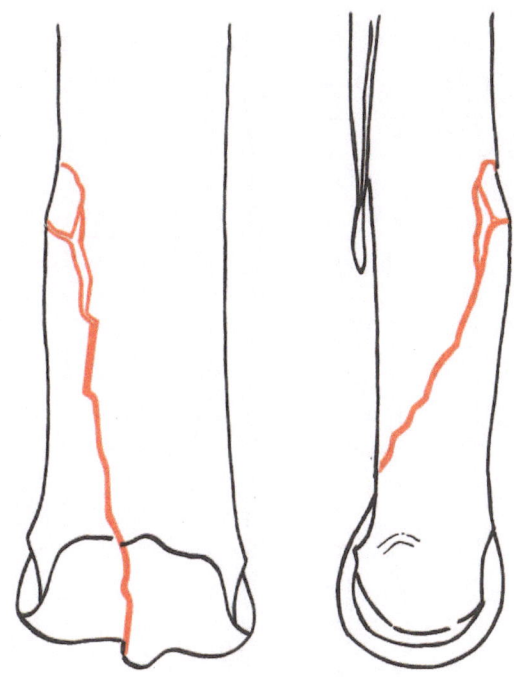

Fig. 4.21

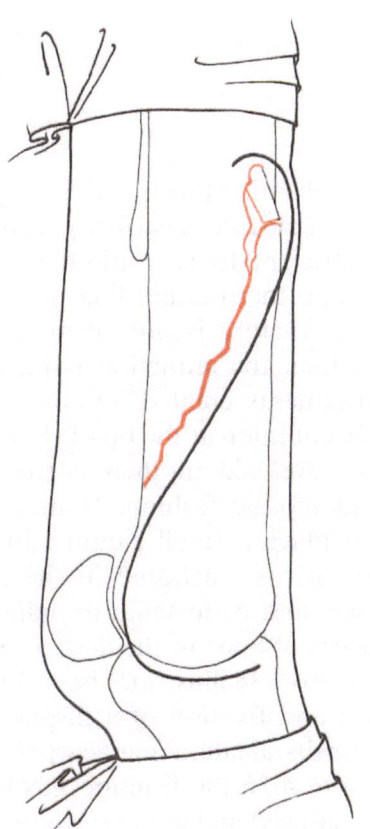

Fig. 4.22

45

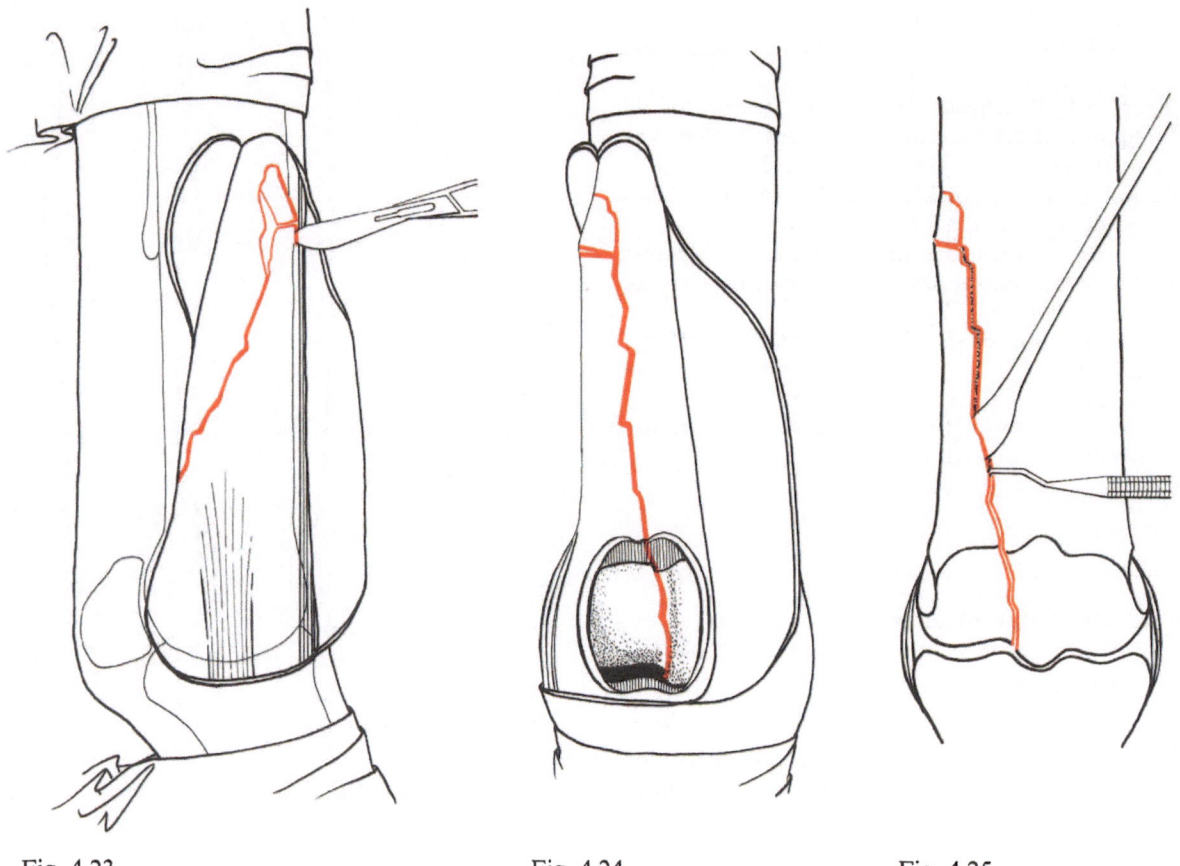

Fig. 4.23   Fig. 4.24   Fig. 4.25

direct visualization through the arthrotomy, the articular surface is perfectly realigned. It is not sufficient to reposition one or two points along the fracture line. If *any* point along the fracture is *not* accurately repositioned, then the reduction is inadequate. Small fragments created by comminution, especially common at the tip of the condylar fragment, are laid in their corresponding defects in mosaic fashion. It may be necessary to place a small catgut suture over these fragments, anchored in the adjacent deep fascia and periosteum to maintain the small pieces of bone in the desired position. Figures 4.26–4.36 illustrate the technique of reduction and fixation of a displaced fracture of the distal lateral metacarpal condyle.

In Figure 4.26 the fracture has been accurately reduced and maintained in position by the placement of two C-clamps. The first clamp is placed through a stab incision in the lateral collateral ligament at the level of the epicondylar fossa. The second clamp is placed 25–30 mm proximal to the first. As the C-clamps are tightened, the fracture plane is placed under compression. Radiographic examination at this point will assure the surgeon of the quality of the reconstruction and the accuracy with which the reduction instruments have been placed. Given positive findings, the distal 4.5 mm clearance hole is drilled through the condylar fragment. Measurements taken during drilling will ensure that the clearance hole has at least reached the fracture plane. Given the size and character of the bone involved, it is probably better to actually cross the fracture plane, thus shortening the length of the pilot hole and reducing the frictional resistance to subsequent tightening of the screw.

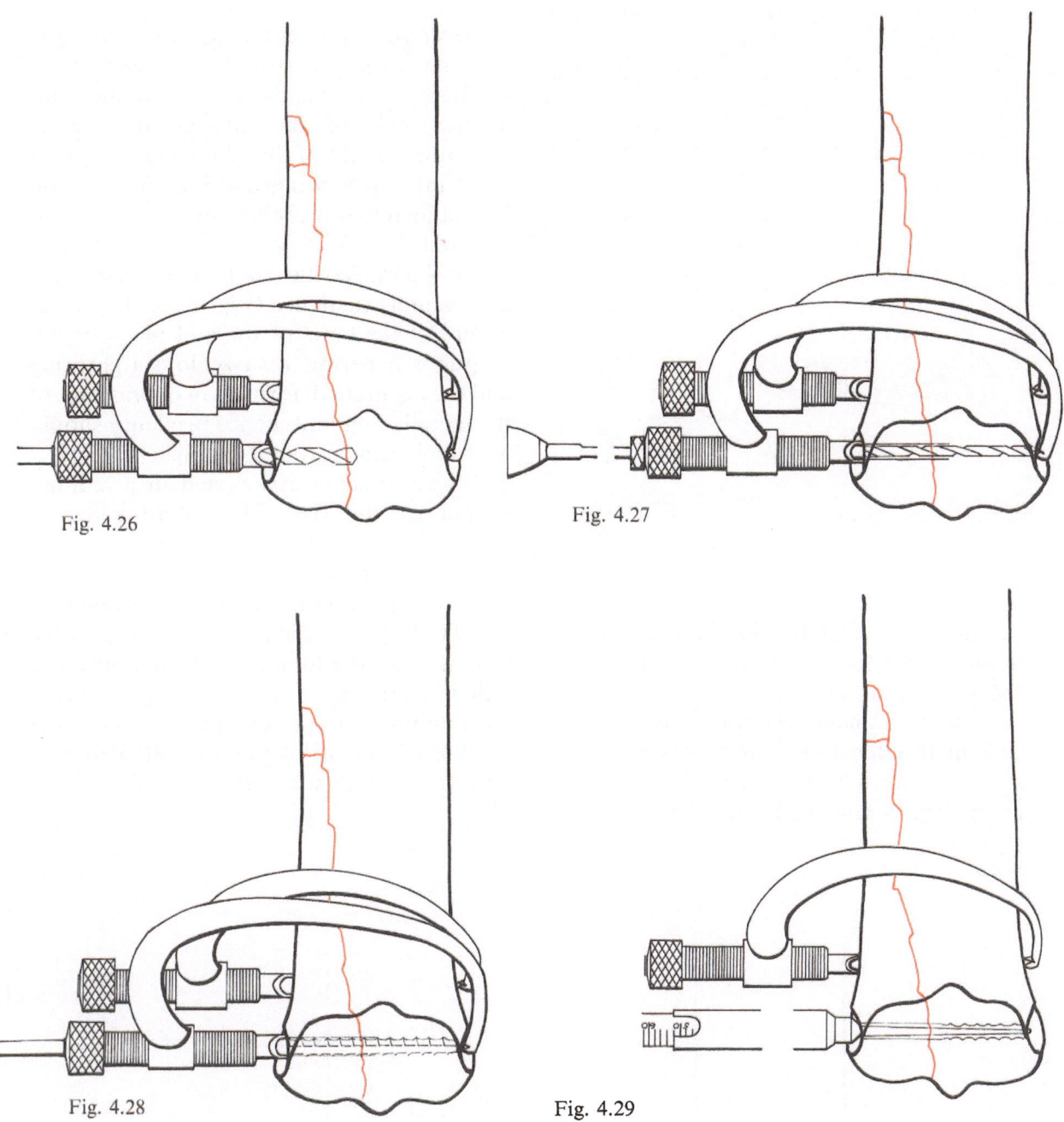

Fig. 4.26

Fig. 4.27

Fig. 4.28

Fig. 4.29

The 3.2 mm sleeve is placed in the guide portion of the C-clamp, and the pilot hole is prepared in the parent portion of the bone (Fig. 4.27). The diameter of the bone at this level in most adult horses will require that the 70 mm drill bit be employed.

The tap is inserted through the guide portion of the C-clamp, and threads are cut in the pilot hole (Fig. 4.28).

The depth gauge is used to determine the appropriate length of screw to be inserted (Fig. 4.29). Note that this step is "out of order" compared with standard procedures in that threads have been cut prior to measurement. The desire to maintain accurate reduction with the C-clamp in place until tapping is complete prevents measurement in the usual sequence. One must be

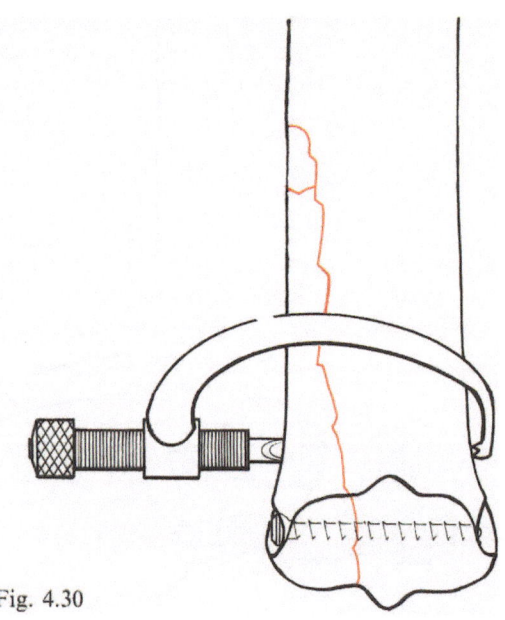

Fig. 4.30

instrument inflicts too much damage upon the overlying collateral ligament. Allowance is made for soft tissues interposed between the base of the depth gauge and the bone as the scale of the instrument is read. The threaded tip of the screw must not protrude into the substance of the opposite collateral ligament if racing soundness is to be restored.

The 4.5 mm cortical bone screw is inserted and securely tightened (Fig. 4.30). The dense nature of the bone of the end of the metacarpus will permit over-zealous tightening and the resultant deformation or breakage of the metallic implant, hence prudence should be exercised as torque is applied.

A second screw is inserted in a manner similar to the first. If a third screw is required, it is usually inserted without the aid of a C-clamp using only the 4.5 mm tap sleeve as a guide (Fig. 4.31). The 4.5 mm hole tends to be perpendicular to the plane of the fracture and the long axis of the bone. The hole is carried into the medullary cavity, as the compressed fracture plane is not perceptible during drilling and insufficient penetration could result in negation of the "lag" effect.

careful not to catch the tip of the instrument in one of the threads, potentially damaging the bone and resulting in an erroneously short measurement. The use of the countersink in this location is unnecessary as the surface of the bone is sufficiently concave to accept the screw head, and the use of the

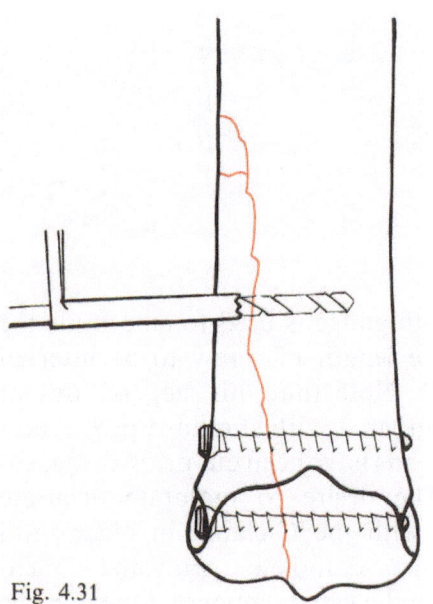

Fig. 4.31

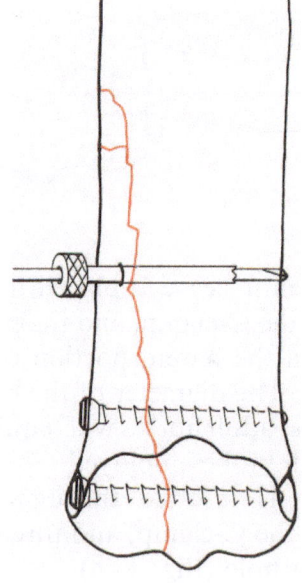

Fig. 4.32

The 3.2 mm drill sleeve is placed in the 4.5 mm clearance hole, and the pilot hole is prepared in the opposite cortex (Fig. 4.32).

The countersink is employed to create a depression large enough to receive the head of the screw (Fig. 4.33).

The depth gauge is used to determine the appropriate length cortical bone screw to be inserted (Fig. 4.34).

Threads are cut in the pilot hole using the 4.5 mm cortical tap (Fig. 4.35).

The third screw is inserted and tightened, placing the entire fracture plane under interfragmentary compression (Fig. 4.36).

Postoperatively, closure is routine using 00 chromic catgut in the deep fascia, periosteum, and fibrous layer of the joint capsule, as well as in the stab incision made in the

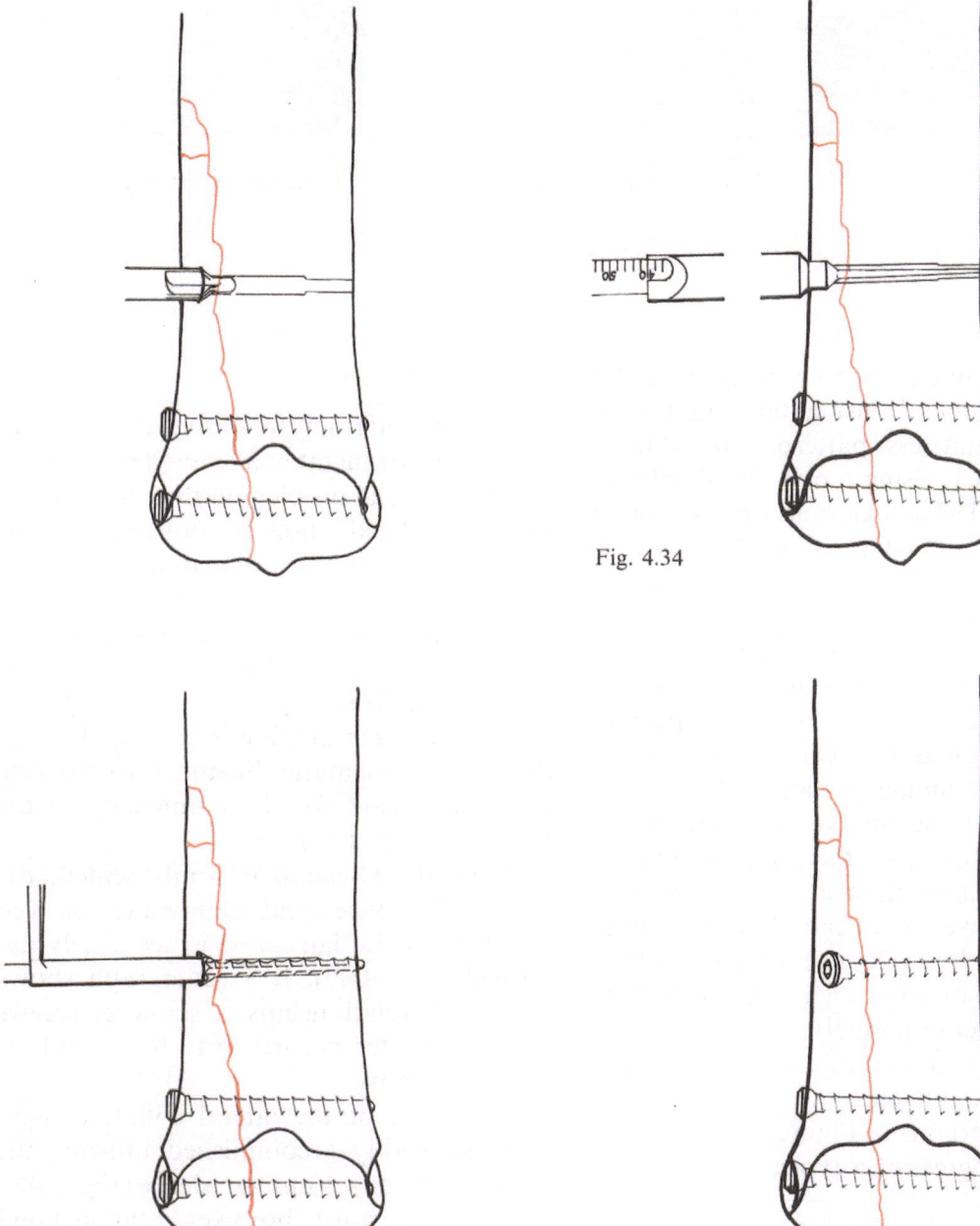

Fig. 4.34

Fig. 4.35

Fig. 4.36

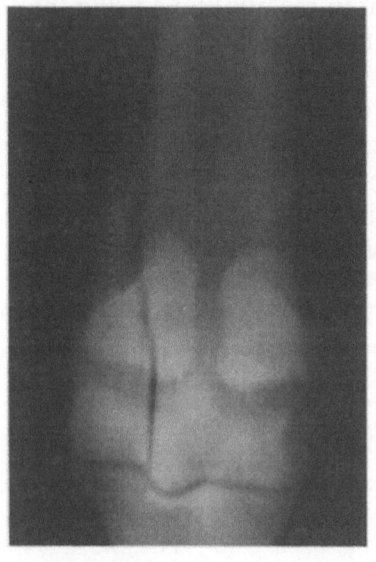 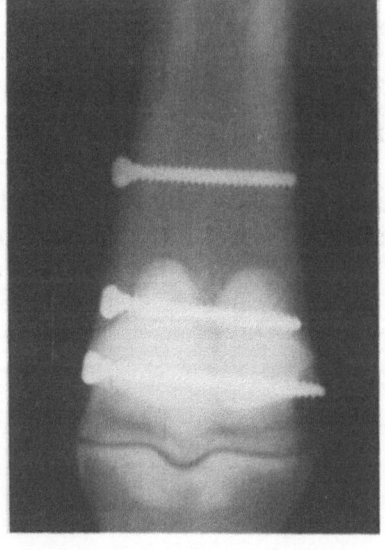 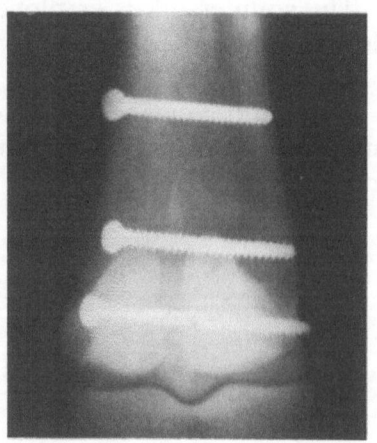

a preoperative   b immediately postoperative   c 12 weeks postoperative

Fig. 4.37 a–c

collateral ligament. A row of subcuticular sutures are placed, using 00 catgut in a horizontal mattress pattern. The skin is closed routinely using a non-absorbable suture material. No external support other than an elastic bandage is employed. For 6 weeks, the animal is stall rested, and for an additional 6 weeks, handwalking exercise is prescribed. Follow-up radiographs are taken 12 weeks after surgery and, given positive findings, the animal is turned out to pasture for an additional 12 weeks before the resumption of training to race.

Similar fractures of the distal metatarsal condyles occur, and their repair may be approached in a manner identical to that described above. Great care should be given, however, to the evaluation of preoperative radiographs, as additional bony pathology located further proximally is common in the hindleg and can seriously compromise the postoperative outcome.

The radiographs in Figure 4.37 a–c document the progress of a typical case.

b) Non-displaced

Non-displaced fractures of the lateral, distal, metacarpal or metatarsal condyles present a simpler surgical problem in that arthrotomy and manual reduction are not necessary to achieve accurate reconstruction.

Figure 4.38 shows a stab incision carried through the skin and lateral collateral ligament to the bone at the level of the lateral epicondylar fossa.

A second stab incision is created through the medial collateral ligament to provide good anchorage for the pointed tip of the C-clamp (Fig. 4.39).

When the C-clamp is firmly seated, the fracture is reduced and the intended path of insertion of the lag screw is accurately described (Fig. 4.40). If a radiograph shows acceptable relationships, a screw or screws may be inserted according to the technique described above.

Protection of the lateral collateral ligament is readily accomplished utilizing the C-clamp or the 4.5 mm tap sleeve (Fig. 4.41). The surgeon must, however, bear in mind that the medial collateral ligament is closely

50

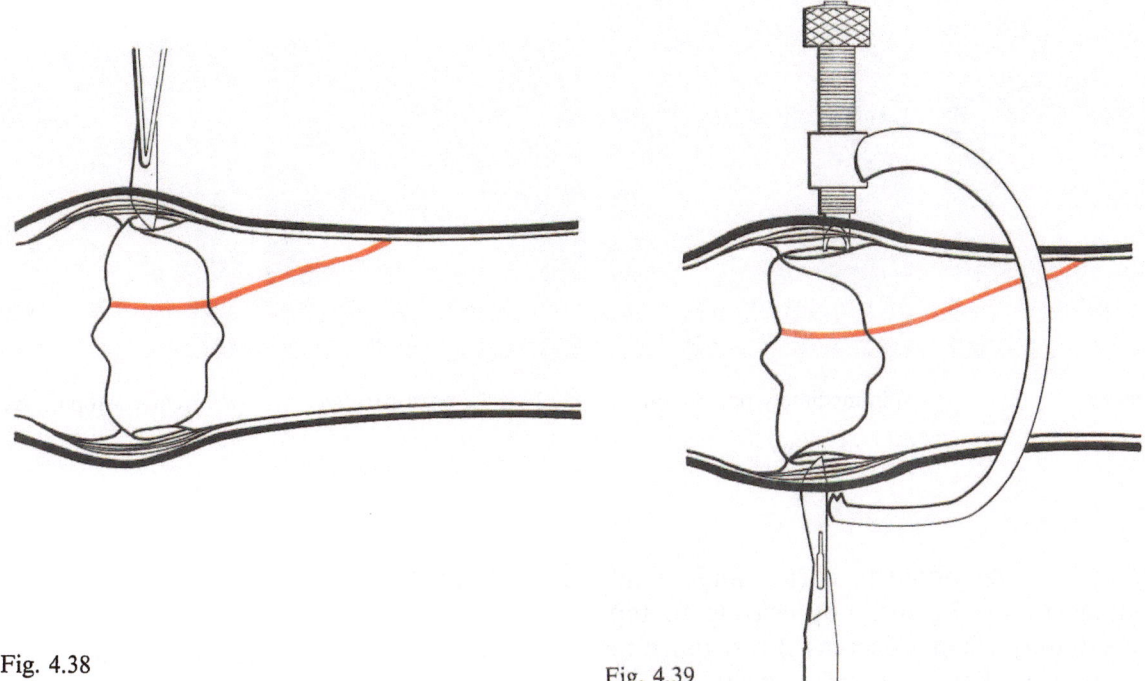

Fig. 4.38

Fig. 4.39

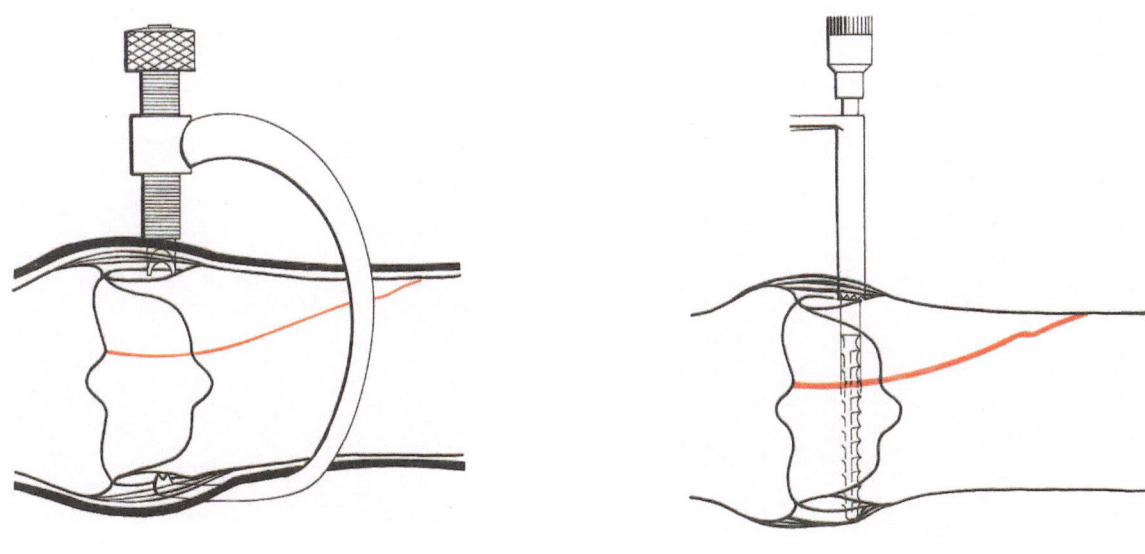

Fig. 4.40

Fig. 4.41

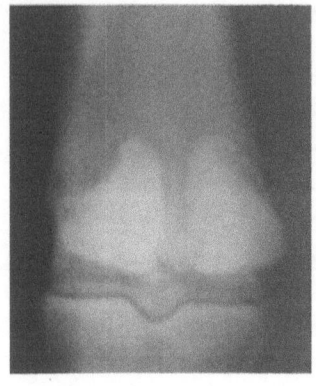 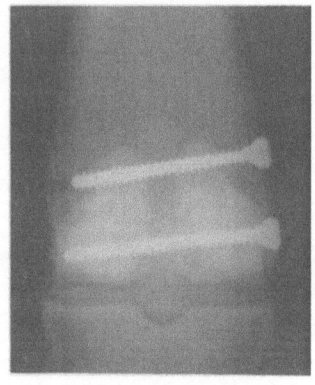 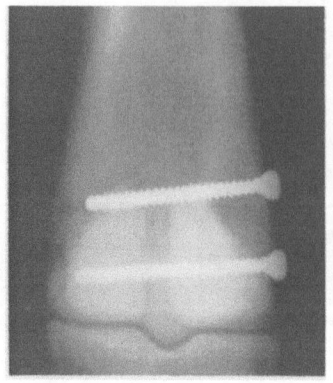 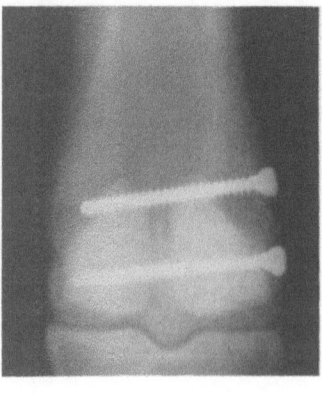

a preoperative   *b* immediately postoperative   *c* 12 weeks postoperative   *d* 1 year postoperative

Fig. 4.42 a–d

applied to the opposite cortex and avoid damage to the ligament by ceasing to tap immediately when a decreased resistance to the passage of the instrument is felt.

The radiographs reproduced in Figure 4.42 a–d document the progress of a typical case.

References

Alexander, JT, Rooney, JR: The biomechanics, surgery and prognosis of equine fractures. Proc. Amer. Assoc. Equine. Pract. *18* (1973): 219–35

Meagher, DM: Lateral condylar fractures of the metacarpus and metatarsus in horses. Proc. Amer. Assoc. Equine. Pract. *22* (1977): 147–54

Rooney, JR: Distal condylar fractures of the cannon bone in the horse Mod. Vet. Pract. *52* (1974): 113.

4.3 Sesamoid Fractures

Mid-transverse fractures of the proximal sesamoids are injuries common in the racing Thoroughbred and Standardbred. Untreated, most of these fractures will go on to form non-unions. By means of lag screw fixation, the tensile stresses to which the bone is subjected may be neutralized to bring about healing. As with any other fracture affecting an articulation, the preoperative radiographs should be carefully evaluated for the presence of degenerative joint disease. Surgery should not be contemplated in those cases with significant pathologic changes as the chances of restoring the horse to racing soundness are small despite good fracture healing.

The *surgical approach* is through a curvilinear skin incision, the proximal arc of which is based posteriorly and centered over the proximal volar outpouching of the fetlock joint, while the distal arc is centered over the base of the affected sesamoid. The distal dissection is carried down to the division between the straight and the oblique sesamoidean ligament. The natural division between these ligaments is followed proximally until the base of the sesamoid is encountered. Proximally, the dissection is carried down to and through the proximal volar outpouching of the fetlock joint in a manner similar to that used for the removal of apical fragments of the proximal sesamoids. With the digital joints in partial flexion, a small stab incision is made from inside the joint into the fibrocartilaginous tissue proximal to the apex of the sesamoid. The ledge so created will serve as a point of

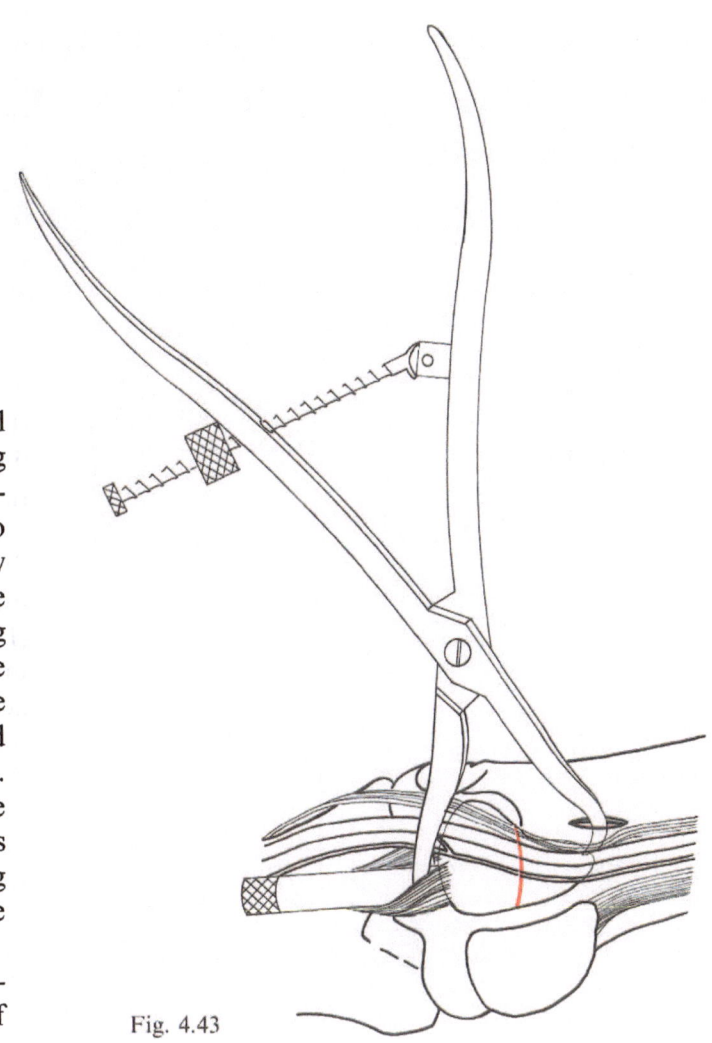

Fig. 4.43

anchorage for the reduction clamp to be placed subsequently.

Figures 4.43–4.47 illustrate the surgical procedure.

The base or guide portion of the bone-holding clamp is slid into the slit created in the oblique sesamoidean ligament until the instrument rests firmly on the base of the sesamoid (Fig. 4.43). The tip of the instrument is introduced into the fetlock joint and placed upon the ledge created proximal to the apex of the fractured bone. The handles of the instrument are squeezed, reducing the fracture, and the configuration is maintained in place by tightening the knurled retention nut. Accuracy of the reduction at the artic-

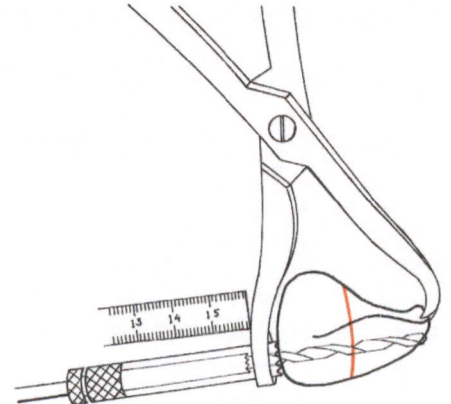

Fig. 4.44

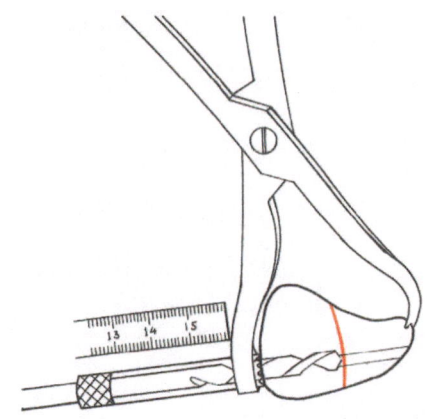

Fig. 4.45

ular surface should be checked by inserting a finger into the flexed fetlock joint. The placement of the clamp may also be checked radiographically at this point.

With 4.5 mm and 3.2 mm sleeves in position, the sesamoid is drilled through from distal to proximal (Fig. 4.44). Measuring the progress of the drill bit will substantiate distances measured on preoperative radiographs and will represent an added safeguard against the placement of an implant of inappropriate length. Flexion of the fetlock joint and inclination of the handles of the reduction forceps abaxially will facilitate introduction of the drill bit.

The 3.2 mm sleeve is removed and the distal portion of the hole is enlarged to 4.5 mm by means of the corresponding drill bit (Fig. 4.45). Measurement during drilling is important so that adequate enlargement is achieved without, at the same time, damaging the pilot hole. The reversed order of drilling in this procedure will help guard against splitting the distal fragment especially in cases where the basal portion of the fracture is thin.

The tap is inserted through the 4.5 mm sleeve, and threads are cut in the pilot hole (Fig. 4.46a). Egress of the tap through the apex of the sesamoid may be felt as a decreased resistance to turning and further progress of the instrument should be avoided to prevent inadvertent damage to the suspensory ligament.

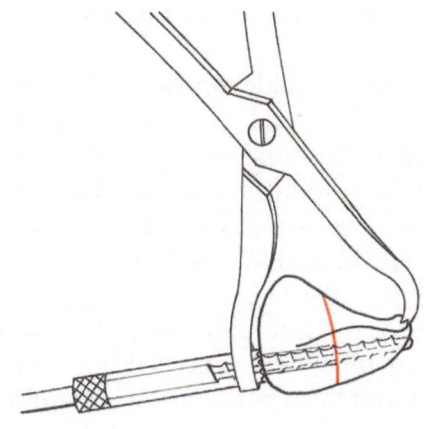

Fig. 4.46 a

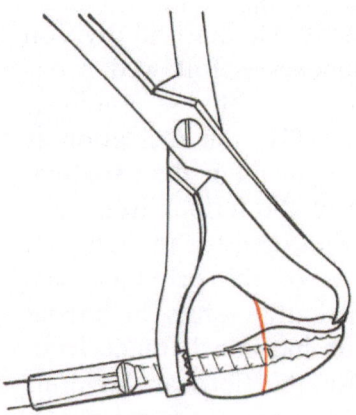

Fig. 4.46 b

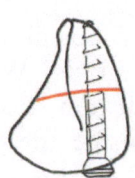

Fig. 4.47

54

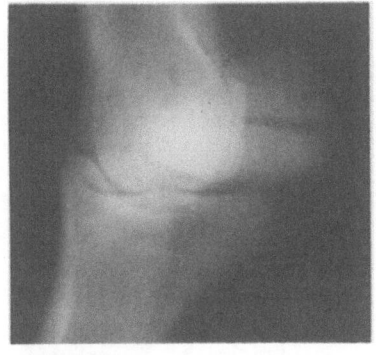 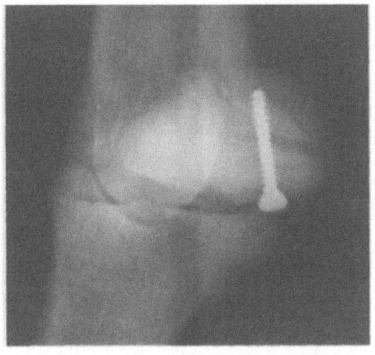 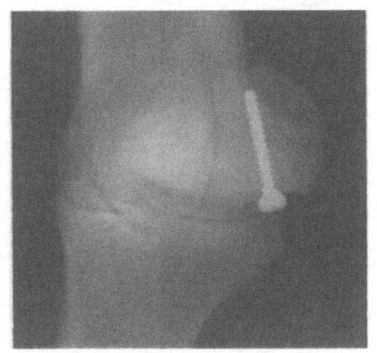

a preoperative   *b* immediately postoperative   *c* 12 weeks postoperative

Fig. 4.48 a–c

Removal of the 4.5 mm sleeve from the guide permits insertion of the screw and shaft of the screwdriver (Fig. 4.46b) facilitating final reduction and fixation before the removal of the clamp.

If the sesamoid clamp has been utilized as described, the screw should emerge just posterior to the true apex of the bone and the direction of the implant should be almost parallel to the sesamoid's axial margin (Fig. 4.47).

Postoperatively, elastic bandages are applied snugly over sheet cotton. The animal is given 6 weeks of stall rest followed by 6 weeks of handwalking or swimming. If 12 week follow-up radiographs show good evidence of healing, exercise in a small paddock is permitted. When facilities and staff are appropriate, we recommend keeping the animal fit by periodic swimming throughout the convalescent period to prevent to some degree the extent of muscle atrophy and flaccidity that inevitably accompany inactivity.

The radiographs in Figure 4.48 a–c illustrate the progress of healing in a typical case.

References

Fackelman, GE: Compression screw fixation of proximal sesamoid fractures. J. Equine Med. Surg. *2* (1978): 32–39

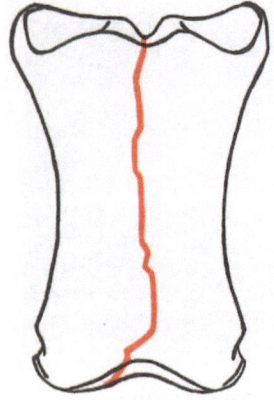 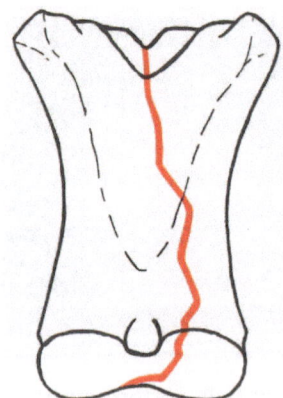 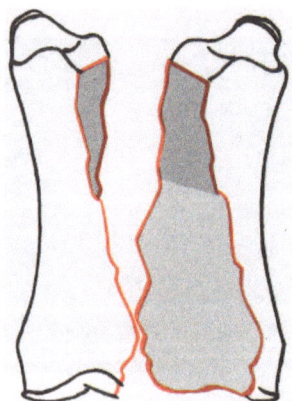

Fig. 4.49

4.4 First Phalangeal Fractures

Sagittal fractures are the fractures of the first phalanx that are most commonly treated by internal fixation. Though the fractures occur more frequently in race-horses, they are also seen in horses used for other purposes. Most sagittal fractures begin at or near the median sagittal groove of the proximal articular surface. They may be incomplete, affecting only that joint surface and the proximodorsal aspect of the anterior cortex. At this stage the fractures are often referred to as "fissures" and may only cause temporary lameness. The minimal radiographic changes may make an accurate diagnosis quite difficult. Complete fractures course through the bone and exit through the medial or lateral cortex just proximal to the attachment of the distal collateral ligament, or they carry on distally to enter the pastern joint. The plane of the fracture may be almost straight sagittal or describe a spiral and divide the distal articular surface frontally (Fig. 4.49).

The *surgical approach* to the typical first phalangeal fracture is through stab incisions. Since displacement along the fracture line is usually minimal and articular "steps" are uncommon, open reduction is not necessary. In fact, over zealous efforts at reduction seem contraindicated owing to the inevitable damage done to overlying soft-tissue elements. The extensor branches of the suspensory ligament, the proximal condyles or "wings", the common digital extensor tendon, the distal condyles, and the borders of attachment of the distal sesamoidean ligaments all serve as good landmarks to assist in the correct placement of implants relative to the fracture plane. All of these landmarks are readily palpable through the skin.

Figures 4.50–4.58 illustrate the surgical procedure.

A point is selected approximately 10 mm anterior and proximal to the branch of the suspensory ligament where it crosses over the first phalanx (Fig. 4.50). This will be the point of insertion for the proximal, subarticular screw. From this position, if drilling is carried out perpendicular to the long axis

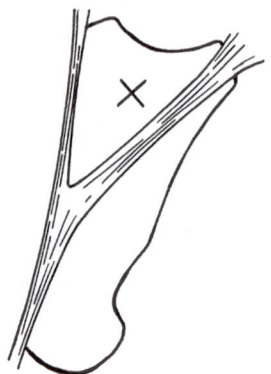

Fig. 4.50

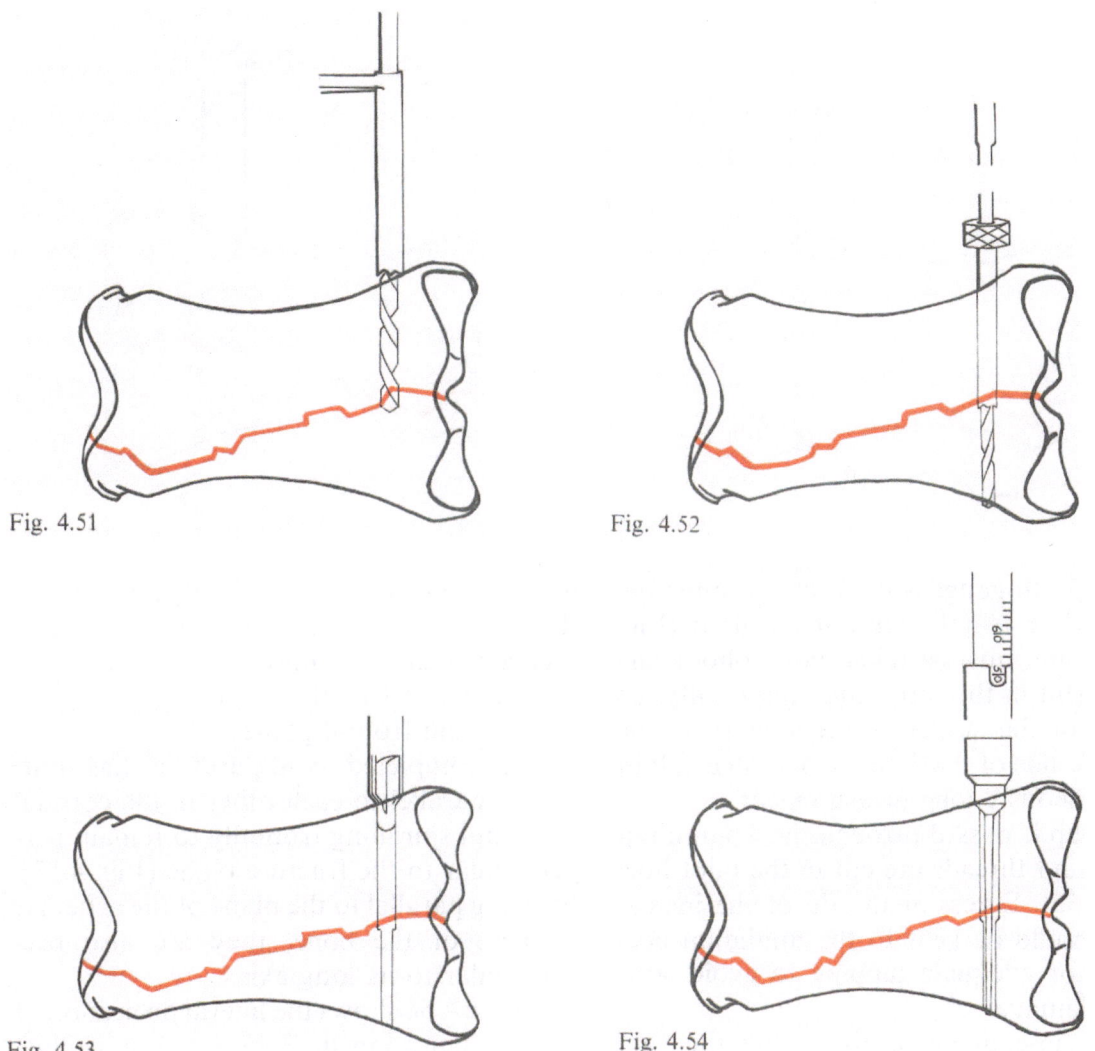

Fig. 4.51

Fig. 4.52

Fig. 4.53

Fig. 4.54

of the limb, the median sagittal groove of the proximal articular surface will not be endangered.

Through the corresponding tap sleeve, a 4.5 mm clearance hole is prepared in the cortex nearer the surgeon (Fig. 4.51). Care is taken either by intraoperative radiography or linear measurement to assure that the clearance hole reaches or just crosses the fracture plane. In the dense subarticular bone filling this area of the first phalanx, it is difficult or impossible to detect the minimally displaced fracture through differences in drilling characteristics.

The 3.2 mm drill sleeve is placed in the 4.5 mm clearance hole, and the pilot hole is prepared in the opposite cortex (Fig. 4.52). Care must be taken not to allow excessive egress of the 3.2 mm drill bit through the opposite cortex, as damage to the periosteum and the opposite extensor branch of the suspensory ligament may result.

The countersink is used to prepare a depression that will accept the head of the screw (Fig. 4.53). Adequacy of countersinking becomes especially important when the axis of a screw is not perpendicular to the adjacent surface of the bone. In such cases, the head of the screw may strike one side of the hole before the other, and as the screw is tightened, bending and serious weakening of the implant may occur.

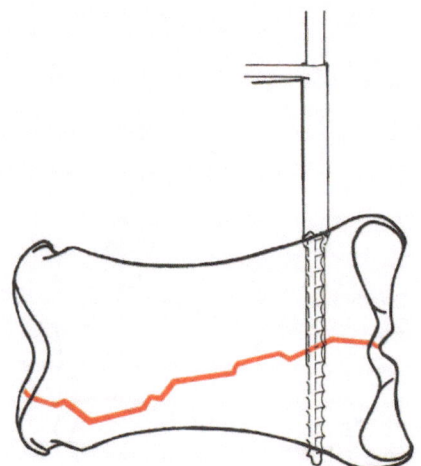

Fig. 4.55

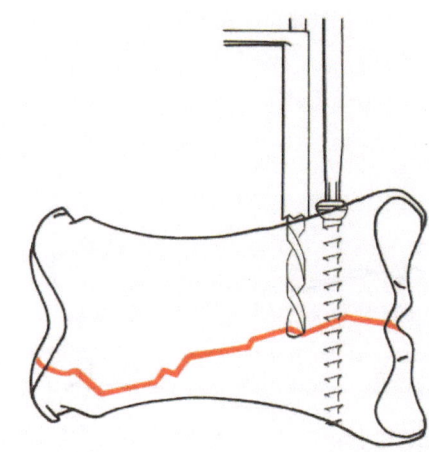

Fig. 4.56

The depth gauge is used to determine the appropriate length screw to be used (Fig. 4.54). Care must be taken not to hook the instrument in the soft tissues (especially the branch of the suspensory ligament) on the opposite side of the bone as this will result in an erroneously long measurement.

The tap is passed through the 4.5 mm tap sleeve, and threads are cut in the pilot hole (Fig. 4.55). Egress of the tip of the instrument should be kept to the minimum necessary for adequate tapping to avoid soft-tissue damage.

After inserting and tightening the first screw, the screwdriver is placed in the screw head and acts as a guide for the insertion of the second screw (Fig. 4.56). In this case, the clearance hole has been prepared approxi-

mately 10 mm distal and slightly posterior to the branch of the suspensory ligament in such a way that the shaft of the second screw will be parallel to that of the first in both coronal and frontal planes.

The completed configuration has four screws parallel to each other in the coronal plane but spiralling frontally to remain perpendicular to the fracture plane (Fig. 4.57). By being parallel to the plane of the articular surfaces of the bone, they are also perpendicular to its long axis.

Figure 4.58 shows the lateral projection of the configuration in Figure 4.57 and illustrates better the orientation of the first two screws relative to one another. The third and fourth screws were placed just abaxial to the common digital extensor tendon. The tips of

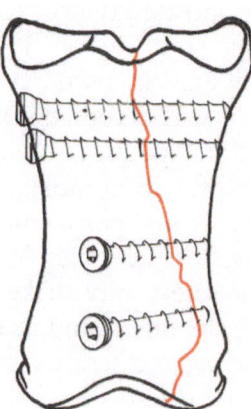

Fig. 4.57

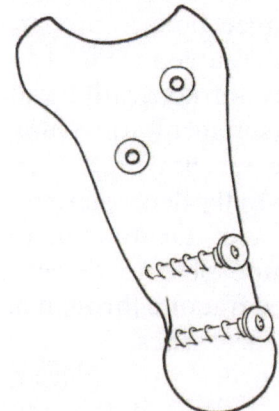

Fig. 4.58

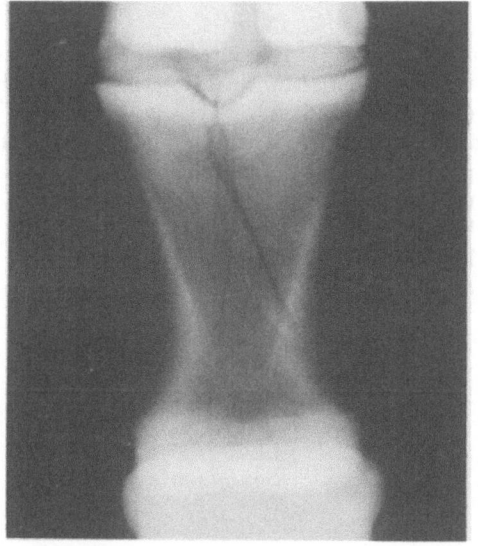

a preoperative

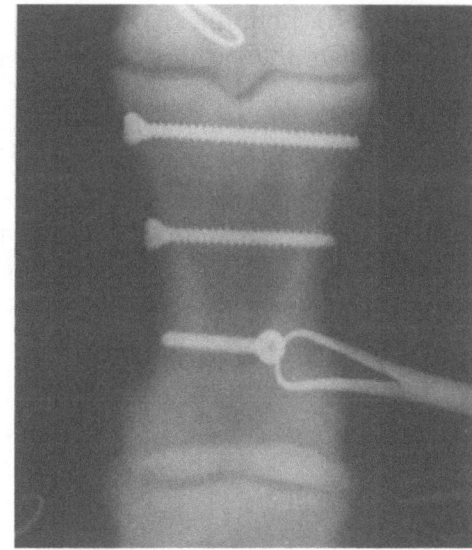

b immediately postoperative

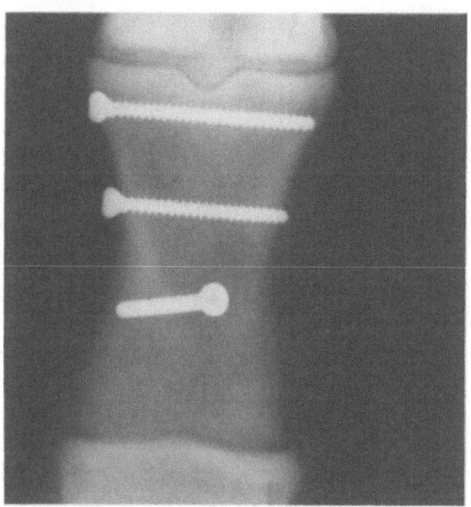

c 12 weeks postoperative

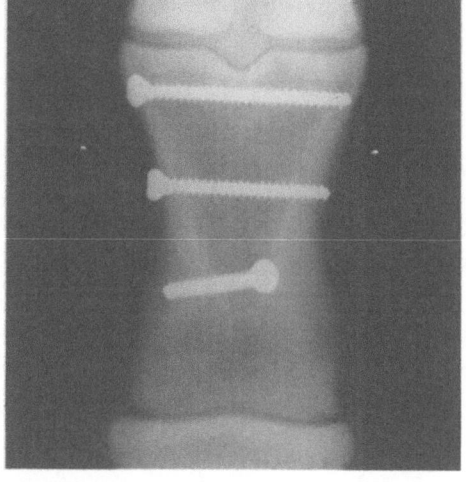

d 1 year postoperative

Fig. 4.59 a–d

these more distally located screws exit abaxial to the border of the distal sesamoidean ligaments. To assure this placement, a C-clamp drill guide may be used during drilling. While the fourth screw undoubtedly adds to the strength of the fixation it is probably optional as regards the final clinical outcome.

Postoperatively, no cast is applied, the limb being snugly wrapped in elastic bandages to prevent hematoma formation. The horse is given 6 weeks stall rest followed by 6 weeks handwalking exercise. Follow-up radiographs are taken 12 weeks postoperatively, and given positive findings, the animal is allowed an additional 12 weeks exercise at pasture before the resumption of training. If facilities permit, swimming exercise may begin as early as 2 weeks postoperatively, to enhance joint mobility and maintain general condition.

If the horse is a riding horse, light riding can be instituted at about 16 weeks after surgery. Exercise should begin at the walk only and be escalated very gradually over the ensuing 8 weeks. No jumping should be undertaken any earlier than 6 months following surgery.

Figures 4.59 a–d show radiographs of a case operated upon in the fashion described.

References

Bohn, D, Waibl, H: Fractures of the first phalanx in the horse. Berl. Münch. Tierärztl. Wochenschr. *90* (1977): 273–275

Dubs, B, Nemeth, F: Therapy and prognosis of first phalanx fractures. Schweiz. Arch. Tierheilk. *117* (1975): 299–309

Fackelman, GE: Sagittal fractures of the first phalanx (P_1) in the horse. Vet. Med. Small Anim. Clin. *68* (1973): 622–636

4.5 Third Phalangeal Fractures

Mid-sagittal fractures of the third phalanx occur in horses and ponies of all kinds. They are usually the result of external trauma to the hooves incurred when the animal kicks a solid object or lands with force upon an unyielding protuberance. Thus, the mid-sagittal fracture differs in etiology from the "wing" fracture, which is thought to be due to chronic imbalance of the hoof wall and the selective trauma of counterclockwise racing. At first, the fracture line may be radiographically indistinct, but demineralization takes place rapidly in this highly vascular bone so that in seven to ten days the crack may be easily demonstrated. Since these fractures are intra-articular, long periods of instability will lead to the development of osteoarthritis of the distal interphalangeal joint (low ringbone) and chronic lameness. For this reason, and to relieve pain and restore the horse to useful soundness as quickly as possible, surgical intervention is indicated.

The *surgical approach* is through a 14.5 mm opening in the horny wall. Prior to surgery, the hoof is scrupulously cleaned and carefully balanced, and the stratum tectorium is removed by light rasping. The hoof is bandaged in cotton soaked in povidone iodine solution and covered by impermeable plastic and tape. These wraps remain in place for 48 hours. At the time of surgery, an Esmarch's bandage is applied, and the hoof is again scrubbed and given a final preparation from the sole surface to the level of the fetlock joint. An adhesive spray is applied, and the entire foot is encased in a sterile, adhesive transparent plastic drape. The remainder of the limb and the patient's body are covered in conventional sterile cloth shrouds.

The surgical procedure is illustrated in Figures 4.60–4.70. After selecting on a lateromedial radiographic projection, the appropriate point to penetrate the hoof wall midway between the articular surface and the semilunar canal measured on a line parallel to the anterior surface of the bone

(Fig. 4.60), calipers are placed symmetrically across the hoof and this distance is recorded (Fig. 4.61).

The countersink, when held against the sole surface just behind the tip of the frog so that a symmetrical half-moon is produced anterior to the instrument, makes a con-

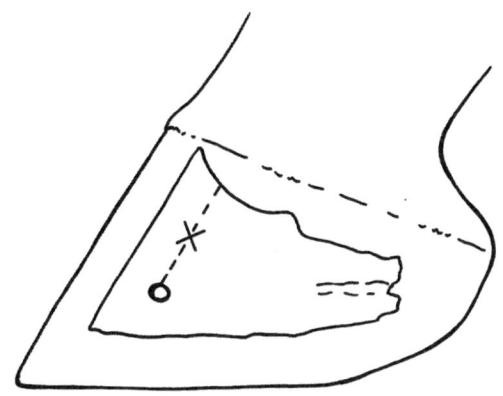

Fig. 4.60

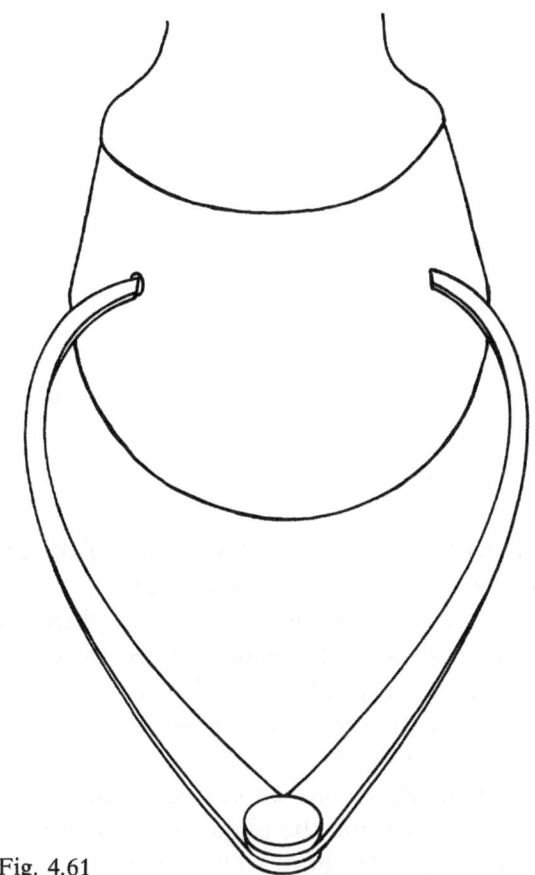

Fig. 4.61

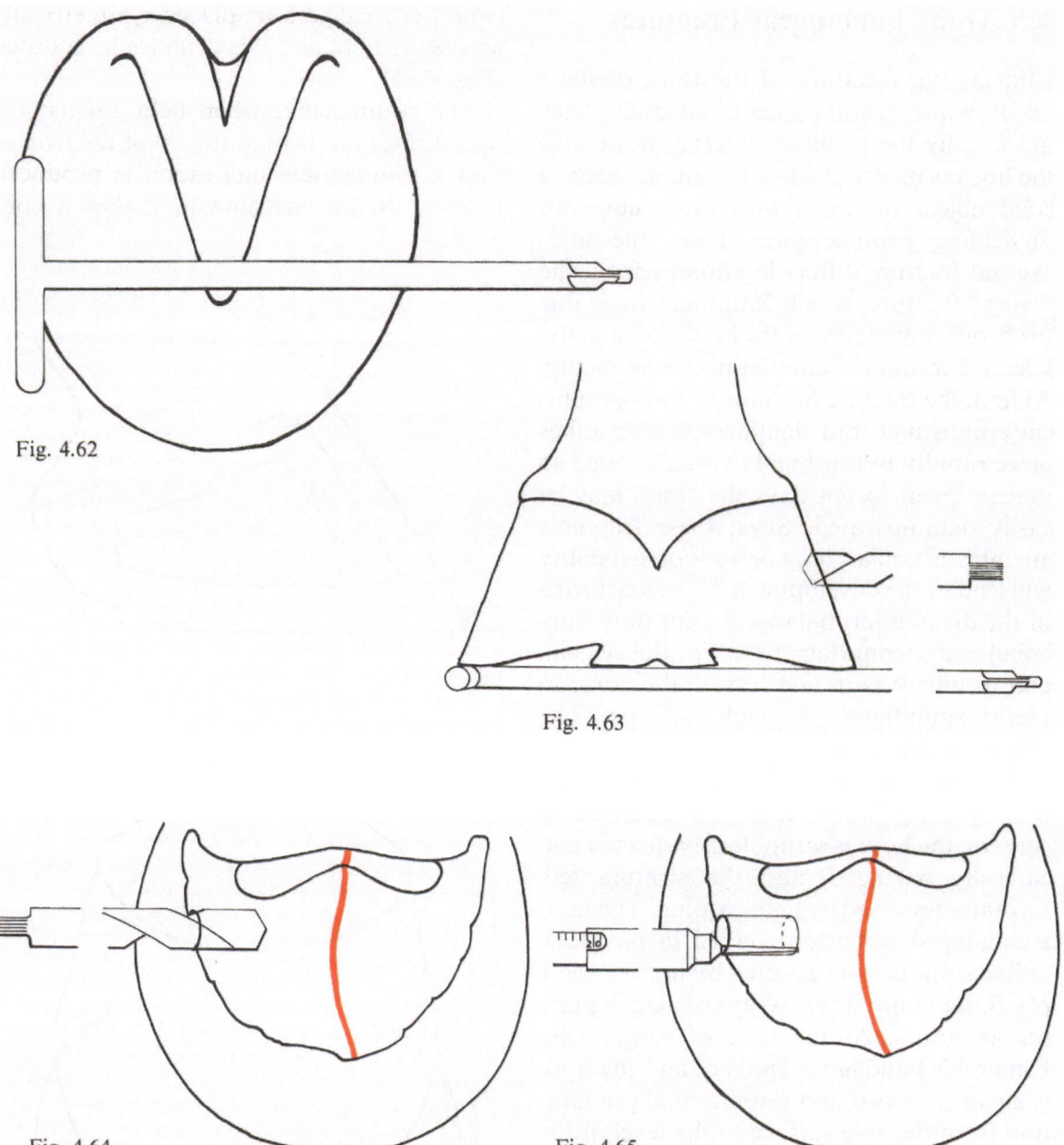

Fig. 4.62

Fig. 4.63

Fig. 4.64

Fig. 4.65

venient guide to direct the course of the drill in the coronal plane (Fig. 4.62).

Since the countersink, when placed as described in the preceding figure, is parallel to the sole, the intrument also acts as a guide to direct the course of the drill in a frontal plane (Fig. 4.63).

Using the point chosen with the aid of radiographs and the planes indicated by the sole surface, the hoof wall is opened utilizing a 14.5 mm drill bit having a shaft diameter of 6 mm (Fig. 4.64).

The depth gauge is used as shown to measure the distance from the surface of the hoof wall to the bone (Fig. 4.65). This measurement is doubled and subtracted from the total measurement of the breadth of the hoof taken with the calipers. The difference represents the exact width of the coffin bone at the level at which the hoof wall was penetrated. The conical shape of the third phalanx renders impossible accurate measurement of this distance from radiographs. Inattention to detail at this point will usually lead to the insertion of implants that are too long. Such screws cause pain due to impingement upon the opposite hoof wall, and the movement of that hoof wall relative to the coffin bone leads to instability, lytic changes along the implant, and the necessity for future removal.

Using the 14.5 mm P_3 tap sleeve, the clearance hole is drilled in the lateral cortex down to the fracture line (Fig. 4.66). Monitoring the distance traversed by the drill bit and comparing these values with a rough estimate made from preoperative radiographs usually permits identification of the fracture line as it is crossed.

The 3.2 mm pilot hole is prepared in the medial cortex (Fig. 4.67). Again, measurement during drilling is helpful in assessing

degree of penetration and allows identification of the medial cortical surface. Drilling is ceased at this point to avoid damage to the sensitive laminae or inadvertent penetration of the medial hoof wall.

Threads are cut in the 3.2 mm pilot hole by means of the 4.5 mm cortical tap (Fig. 4.68). As the instrument exits through the medial cortex, a marked reduction in resistance to turning will be appreciated. Tapping should be discontinued immediately as impacting the tap on the inner surface of the medial hoof wall may strip the threads cut in the bone.

A countersink depression is prepared in the lateral cortex (Fig. 4.69). This depression must be made with care and judgment as the compact bone on the surface of the third phalanx is thin. Over zealous countersinking will result in the head being pulled into the bone as the screw is tightened, thus necessitating the drilling of a new hole at a

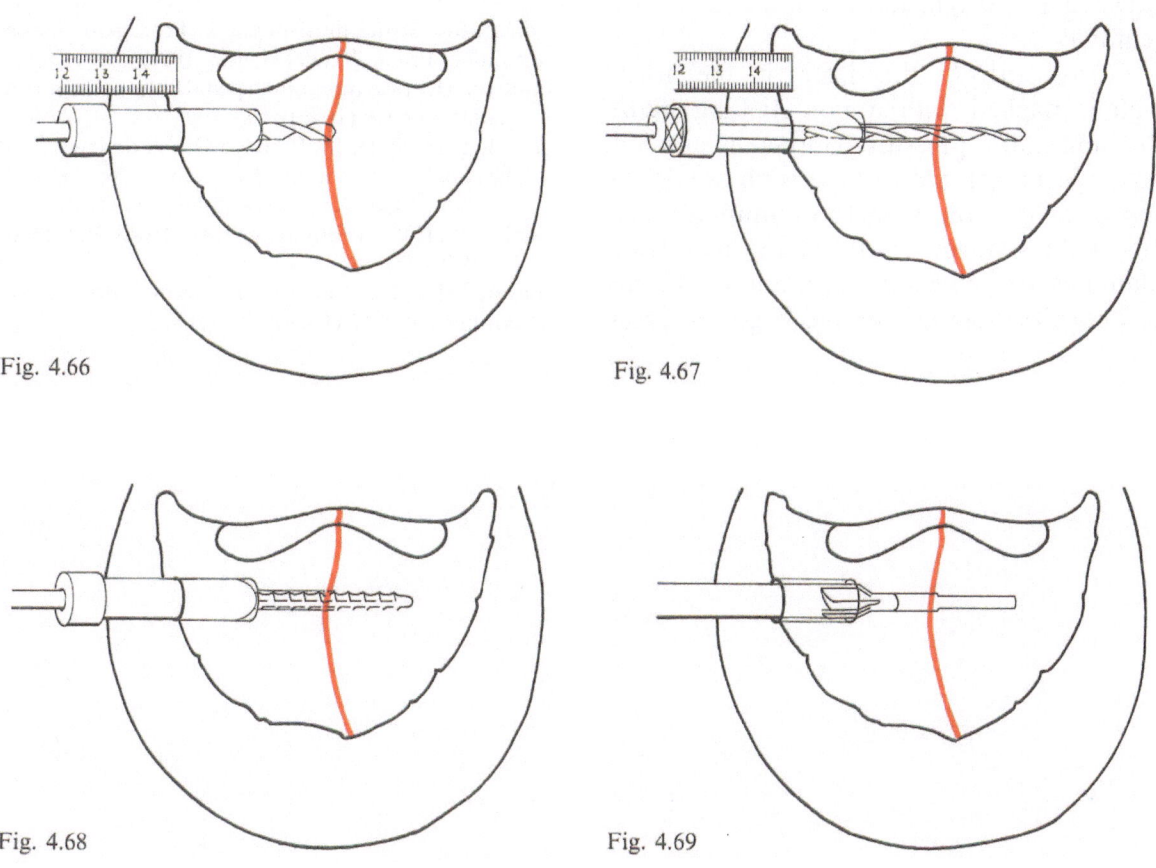

Fig. 4.66

Fig. 4.67

Fig. 4.68

Fig. 4.69

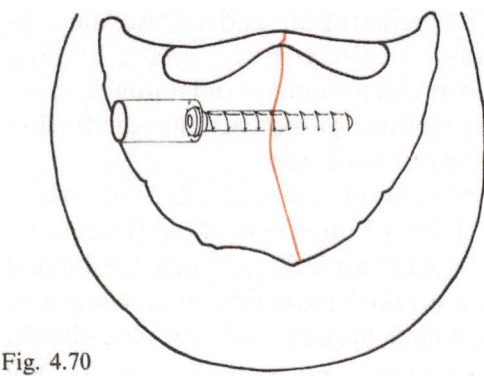

Fig. 4.70

slightly different location or the interposition of a washer beneath the screw head.

The cortical bone screw, when tightened, should compress the fracture line and bear the relationship to the distal margin of the coffin bone depicted in Figure 4.70. Complete radiographic disappearance of the fracture line immediately postoperatively will not be achieved since the hematoma and debris between the fragments are inaccessible for removal.

Postoperatively, the defect in the horny wall is packed with a non-sticking gauze dressing and a pressure bandage is applied. An impermeable plastic boot is placed on the foot as protection against contamination. By 10–14 days postoperatively, the metal implant has been covered by granulation tissue, and cornified epithelium has begun to grow out from the surrounding sensitive laminae. When epithelialization is complete, and the wound is dry, the defect in the wall is patched with an acrylic plastic.

A bar shoe with four stout side clips is applied and the sole is packed with hard acrylic plastic. The horse is given 12 weeks stall rest with the shoe and pack being reset at 4-week intervals. Follow-up radiographs are taken 12–16 weeks postoperatively. Given positive findings the animal is given an additional 8–12 weeks handwalking and pasture exercise before returning to training.

The radiographs shown in Figures 4.71a–d illustrate a typical case before and after surgery.

References

Fackelman, GE: Sagittal fractures of the third phalanx in horses. Vet. Med. Small Anim. Clin. *69* (1974): 1317–1323

Petterson, H: Conservative and Surgical Treatment of fractures of the third phalanx. Proc. Am. Assoc. Equine. Pract. *18* (1972): 183–188

Petterson, H.: Fractures of the pedal bone in the horse. Equine Vet J *8* (1976): 104–109

Scott, EA, McDole, M, Shires, MH: A review of 3rd phalanx fractures in the horse: Sixty-five cases. J. Am. Vet. Med. Assoc. *174* (1979): 1337–1343

Sønnichsen, HV: Fraktur av hovben. Nord. Vet. Med. *15* (1969): 37–44

Weaver, AD: Fracture of the equine pedal bone. Equine Vet. J. *1* (1969): 283–288

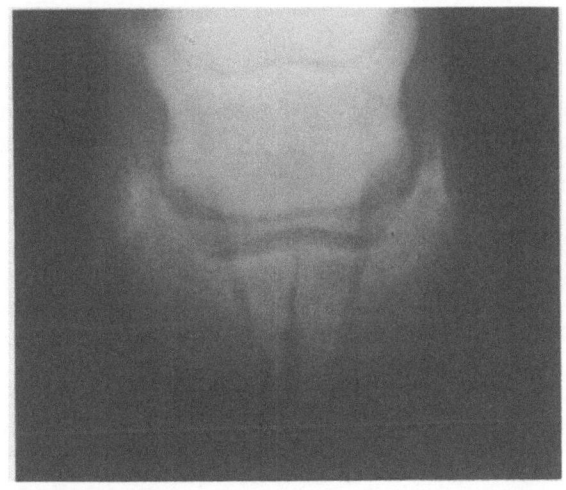

a preoperative

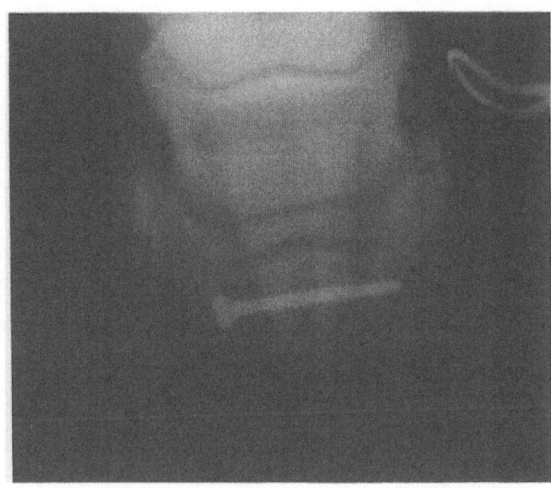

b immediately postoperative

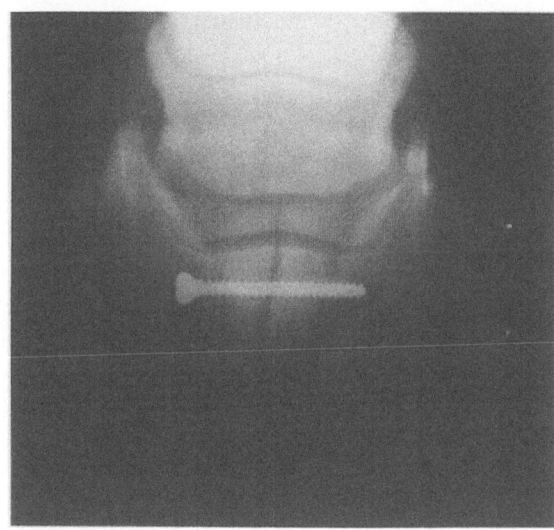

c 12 weeks postoperative

Fig. 4.71 a–d

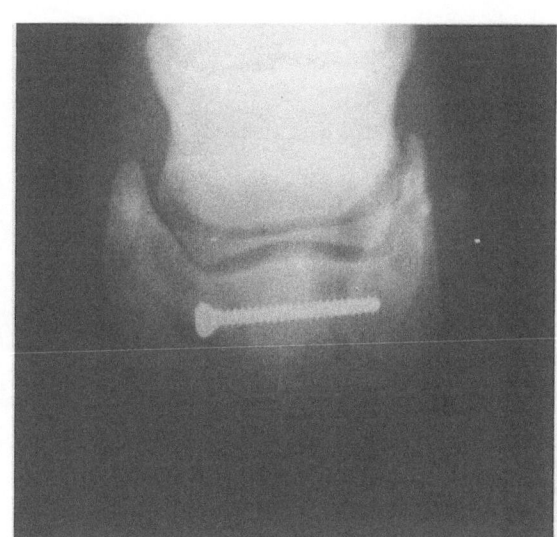

d 28 weeks postoperative

Chapter 5. Plate Fixation

5.1 Olecranon Fractures

Fractures of the olecranon process of the ulna occur due to external trauma to the elbow and are somewhat more common in younger horses, though they also occur in adults. This predilection is due to environmental influences (kicks from other horses, rough play) and not any structural characteristic. The most common fracture splits the ulna transversely through the semilunar notch and thus involves the elbow joint (Fig. 5.1). Without treatment by internal fixation, a non-union results, and the development of osteoarthritis of the radiohumeral joint is inevitable.

The biomechanical situation of the ulna is particularly fortuitous for plating since the bone is constantly under tension. This allows the use of implants of a smaller calibre than would otherwise be practical.

The *surgical approach* to the posterolateral aspect of the ulna is between the muscle bellies of the ulnaris lateralis and the ulnar head of the deep digital flexor. The proximal portion of the skin incision is curved anteriorly so that it does not come to lie directly over the point of the elbow.

Figures 5.2–5.11 illustrate the application of a tension band plate to a typical ulnar fracture.

With the horse in lateral recumbency, the fracture is readily exposed and reduced, and a 3.2 mm hole is drilled approximately 1 cm proximal to the fracture site (Fig. 5.2).

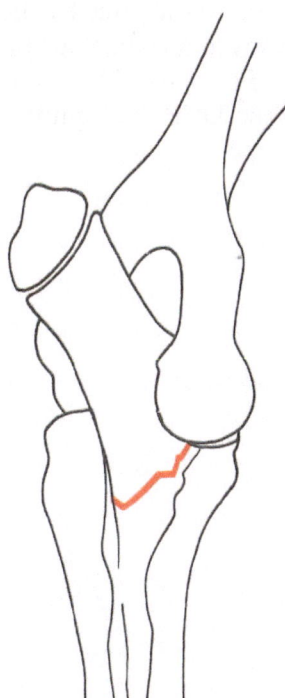

Fig. 5.1

In a young patient (open ulnar growth plate), such as illustrated here, it seems advisable to use cancellous screws at least in the bone of the proximal fragment. Even in an older horse, cancellous bone screws may be needed in the bone proximal to the fracture. The cancellous tap is inserted through the 6.5 mm tap sleeve, and threads are cut in the 3.2 mm hole (Fig. 5.3). The procedure is expedited if a common length for all the screws in the proximal fragment is decided preoperatively based upon measurements from radiographs.

After accurately contouring a narrow dynamic compression plate to conform to the posterolateral aspect of the ulna, the plate is loosely attached to the bone by the insertion of the first screw and is displaced toward the fracture site (Fig. 5.4). The second hole is drilled using the DCP load guide. Drilling is continued until the posterior radial cortex is encountered.

The second hole is tapped in preparation for the insertion of a cortical bone screw (Fig. 5.5). The tap is passed through the 4.5 mm tap sleeve with plate protector in place.

The two screws closest to the fracture are placed eccentrically away from the fracture site (Fig. 5.6). Tightening of these screws will bring about reduction and compression of the fracture according to the dynamic compression principle.

All subsequent screws are placed in the central or neutral position using the corresponding drill guide (Fig. 5.7). With the tightening of each screw, the bone fragments could be potentially moved 0.1 mm closer.

When all screws are inserted and tightened (Fig. 5.8), the fracture should be under

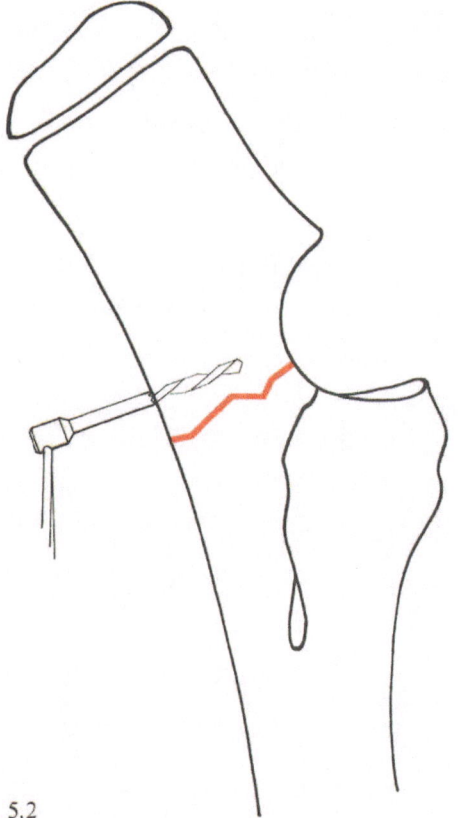

Fig. 5.2

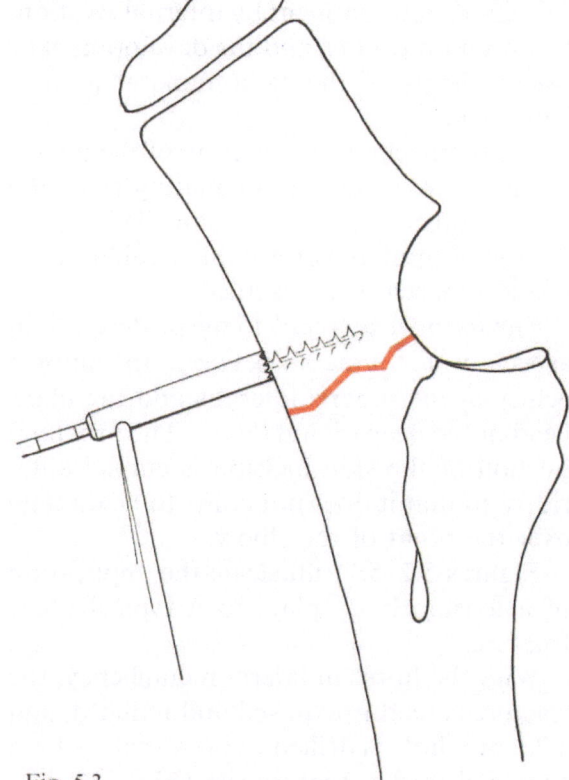

Fig. 5.3

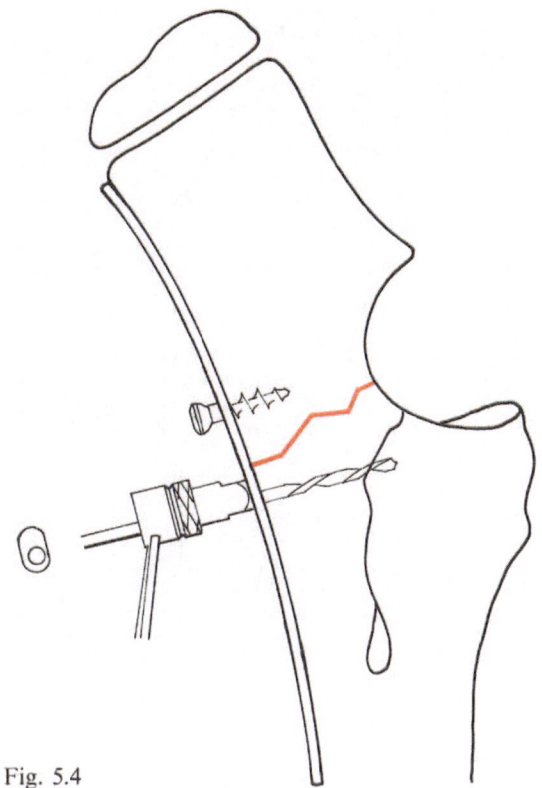

Fig. 5.4

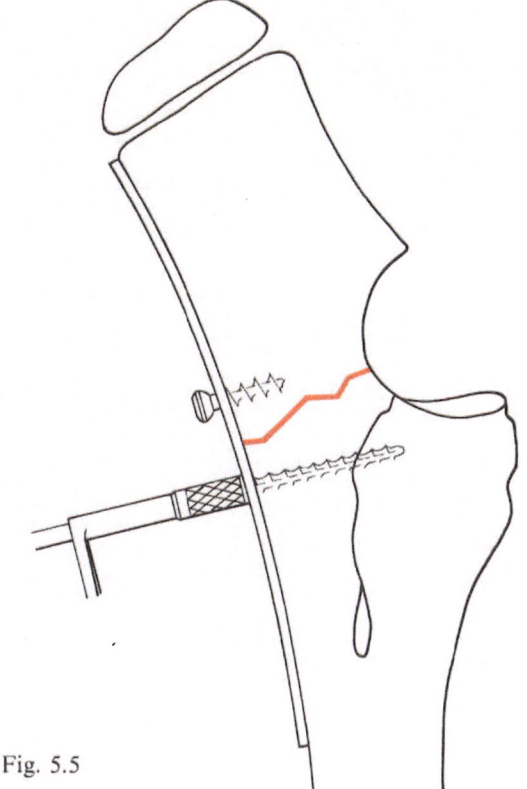

Fig. 5.5

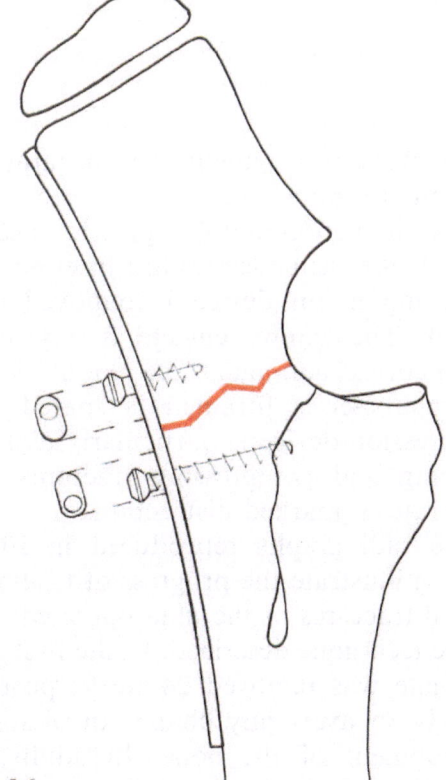

Fig. 5.6

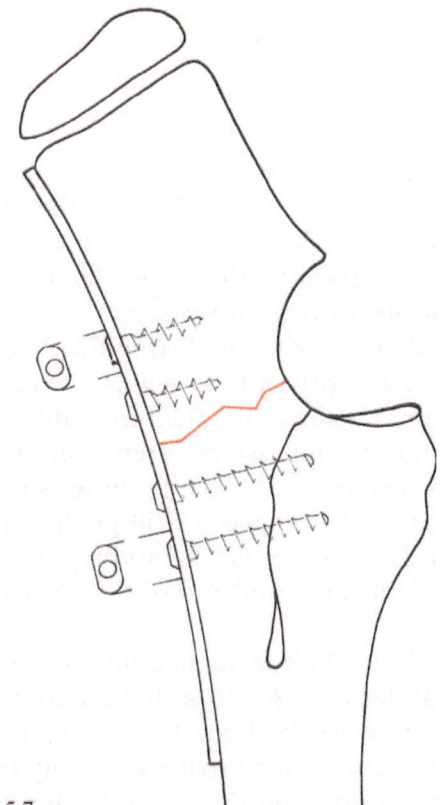

Fig. 5.7

69

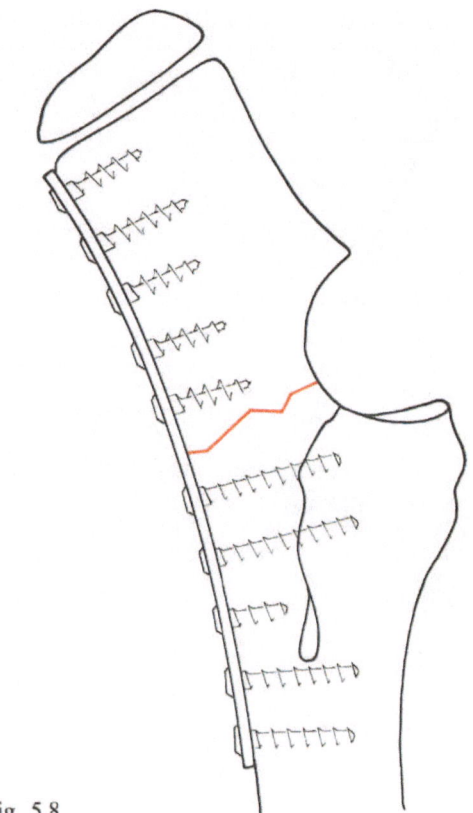

Fig. 5.8

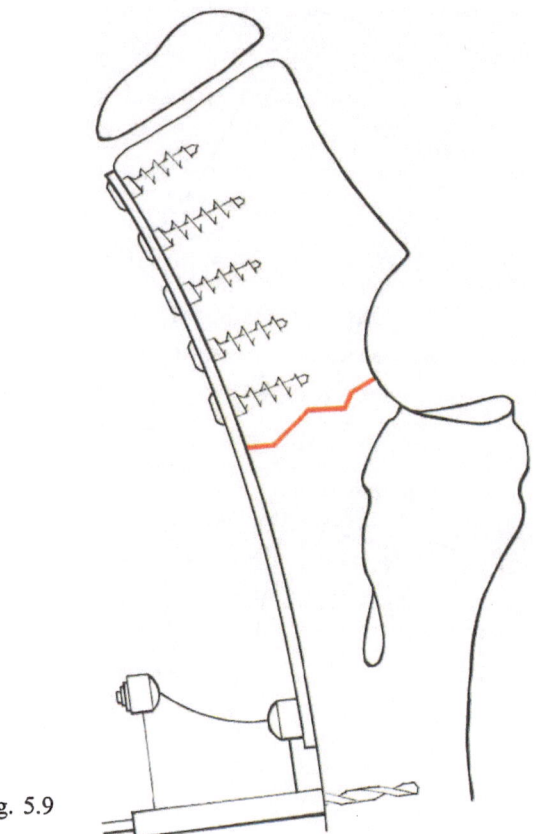

Fig. 5.9

maximum compression. The screw opposite the interosseous foramen between the radius and the ulna should be short in order to prevent damage to the rather large artery that passes through this space.

An alternative to employing the dynamic compression principle to achieve reduction and compression of the fracture is the use of the compression device. Here, all of the screws proximal to the fracture site are inserted, and the special drill guide for the compression device is used to prepare a 3.2 mm hole at the distal end of the plate (Fig. 5.9).

The 3.2 mm hole is tapped and a 4.5 mm cortical screw is used to secure the compression device to the bone (Fig. 5.10 a). The socket wrench is used to provisionally tighten the compression device while alignment of the fracture fragments and accurate reduction are monitored.

With reduction and compression accomplished, the distal screws are inserted, and the compression device is removed (Fig. 5.10 b). The screws engage the posterior radial cortex, and again, the blood vessel in the interosseous foramen is spared. The compression device is particularly useful in reducing and compressing fractures with moderate to marked distraction.

The radiographs reproduced in Figure 5.11 a–j illustrate the progress of healing of typical fractures of the ulna operated upon by the technique described. In the first case, the plate was removed 24 weeks postoperatively to avert any chance of abnormal development of the bone. In adults, the plates are usually left in place.

70

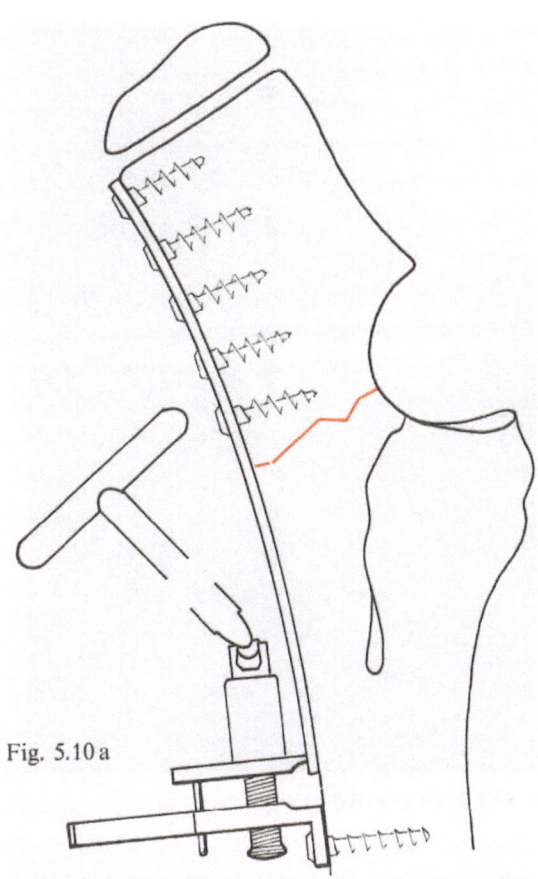

Fig. 5.10 a

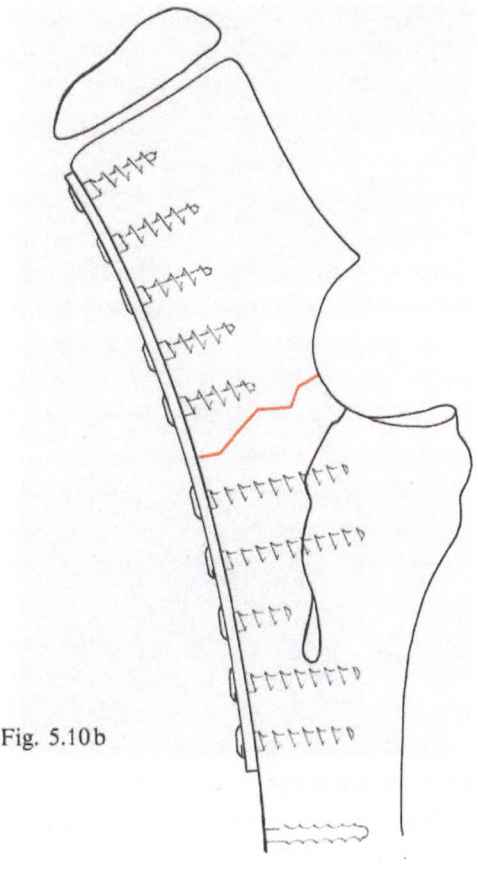

Fig. 5.10 b

References

Fretz, PB: Fractured ulna in the horse. Can. Vet. J. *14* (1973): 50–53

Johnson, JH, Butler, HC: The tension band principle in fixation of an equine ulna fracture. Vet. Med. Small Anim. Clin. *66* (1971): 552–556

Monin, T: Repair of physeal fractures of the tuber olecranon in the horse using a tension band method. J. Am. Vet. Med. Assoc. *172* (1978): 287–290

Scott, EA: Tension band fixation of equine ulna fractures using semi-tubular plates. Proc. Am. Assoc. Equine Pract. *22* (1976): 167–168

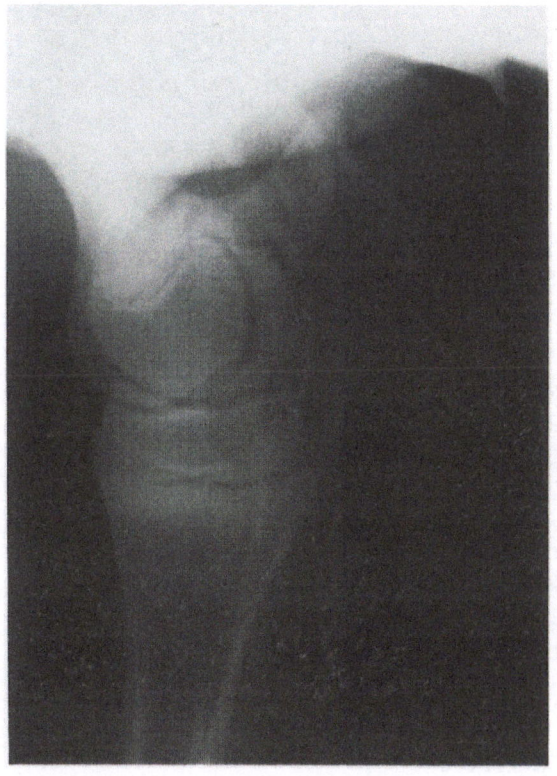

Fig. 5.11 a preoperative

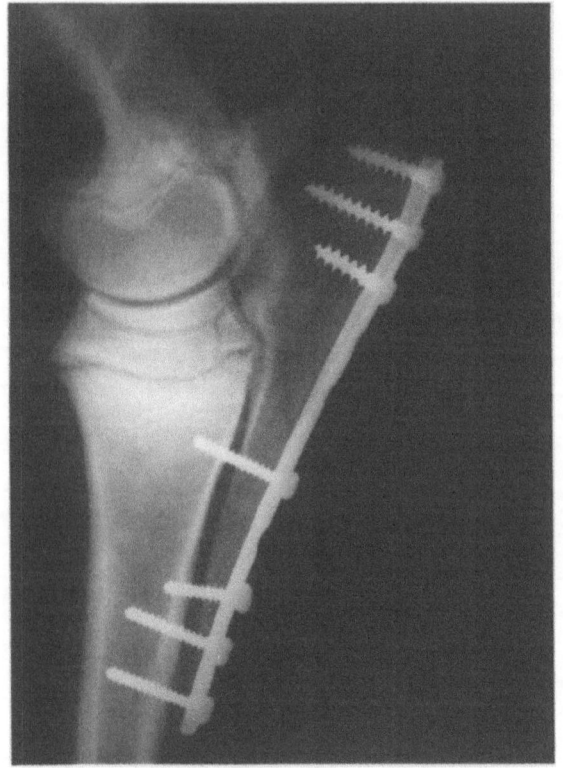

b immediately postoperative

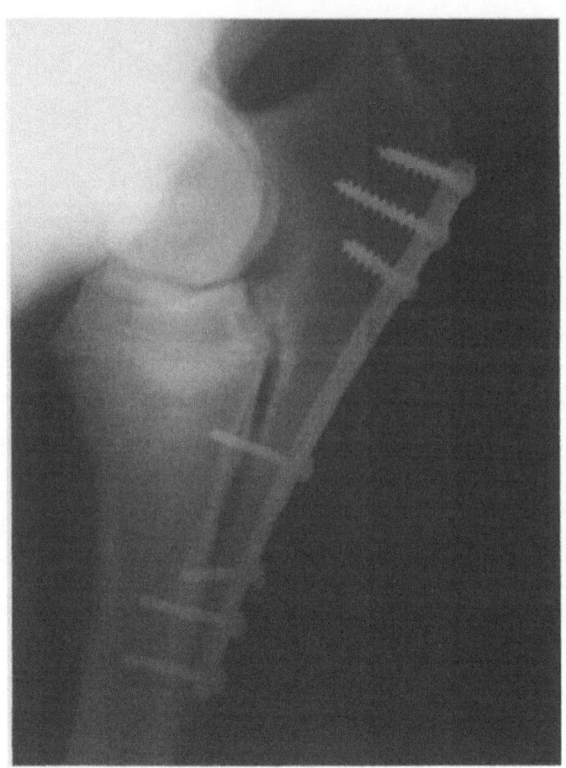

c 6 weeks postoperative

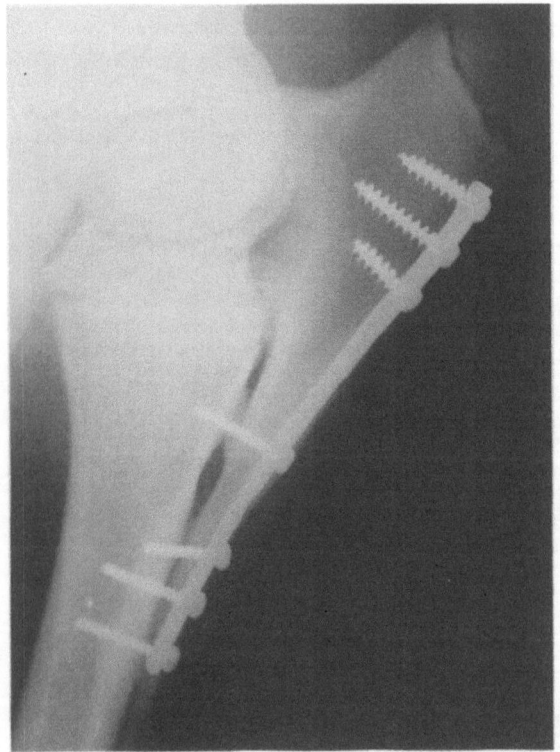

d 12 weeks postoperative
Fig. 5.11 b–e

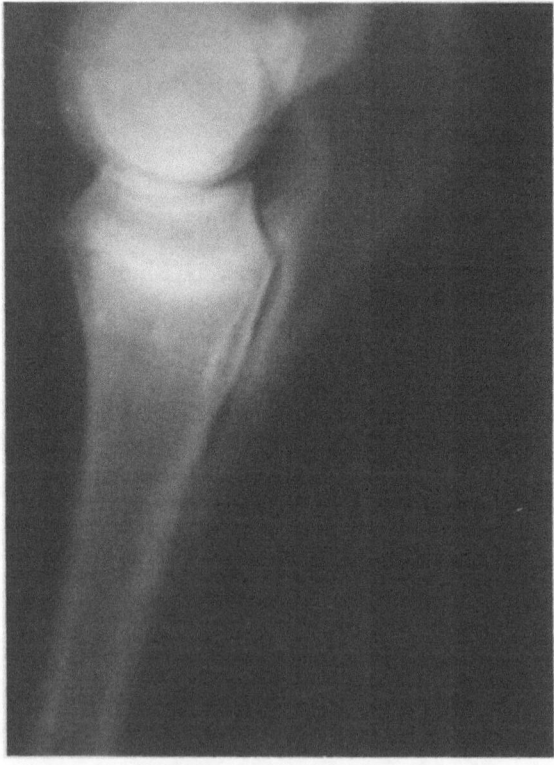

e 24 weeks postoperative (plate removal)

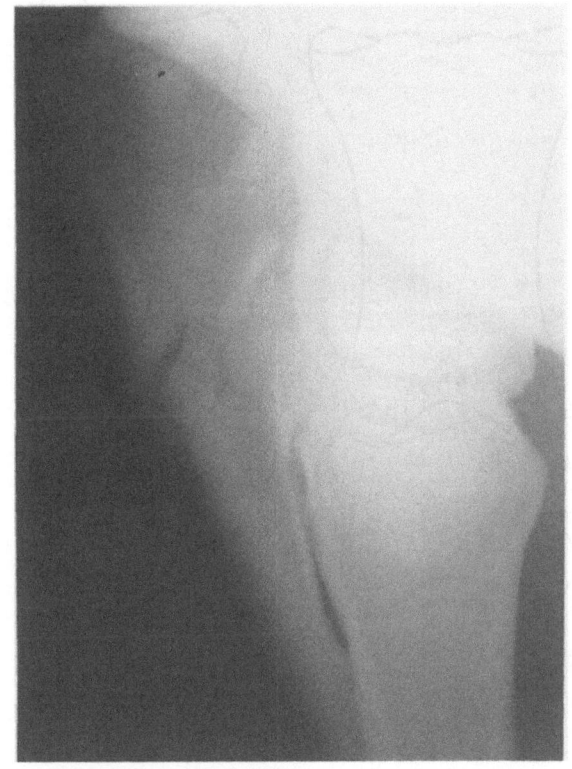

f preoperative (non-union)

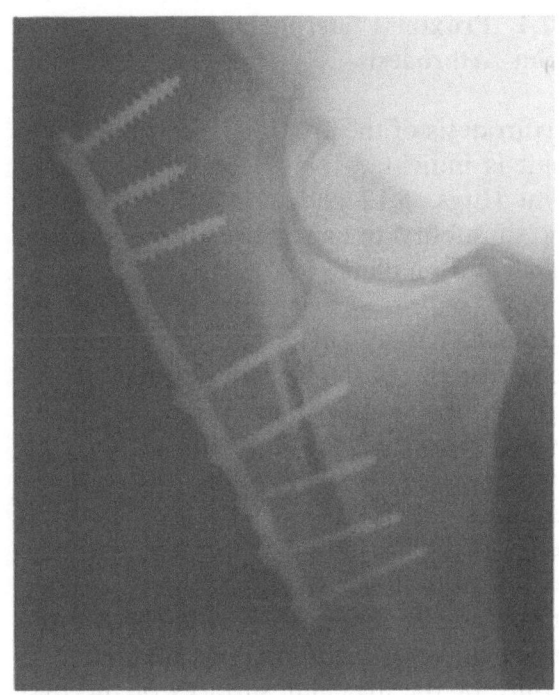

g immediately postoperative

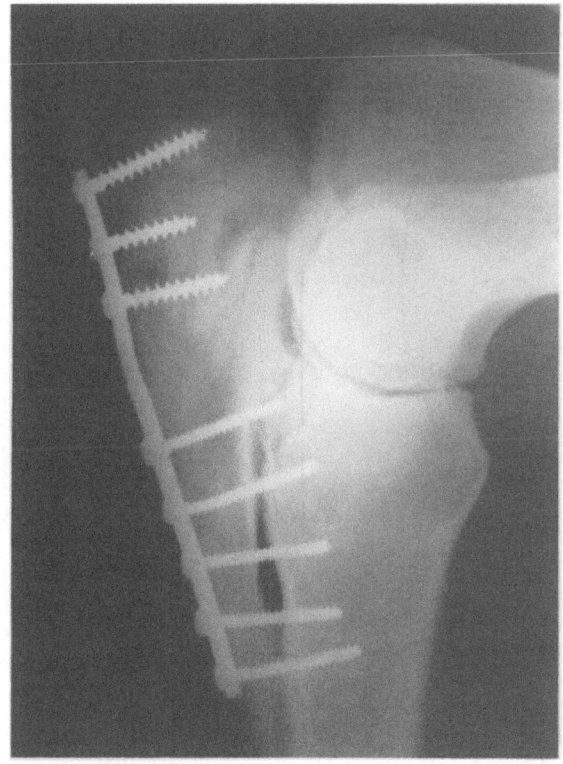

h 12 weeks postoperative
Fig. 5.11 f-i

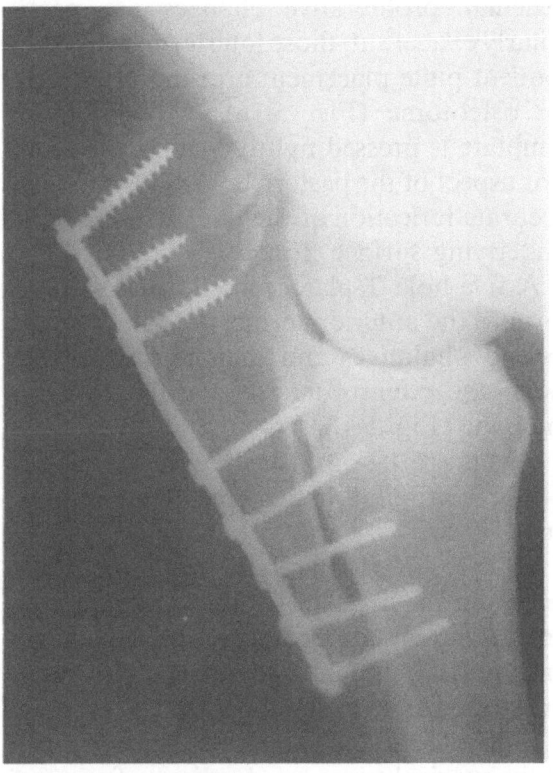

i 24 weeks postoperative

5.2 Arthrodeses

5.2.1. Proximal Interphalangeal Joint Arthrodesis

Arthrodesis of the proximal interphalangeal joint is indicated for osteoarthritis of that joint (Figs. 5.12 and 5.13) as well as for certain subluxations and fractures of the first or second phalanges.

The *surgical approach* is through an inverted Y-shaped skin incision on the anterior aspect of the pastern extending distally almost to the coronary band (Fig. 5.14). After reflection of the skin flaps thus produced a simple split, or where more exposure is required, a Z-plasty of the extensor tendon is performed. The joint capsule is incised coronally, and this incision is carried to the origin of the suspensory ligament of the navicular bone. This permits adequate exposure of the articular surfaces of the first and second phalanges to provide for removal of the articular cartilage (Fig. 5.15). If periarticular proliferative changes are particularly exuberant, those interfering with subsequent plate placement are smoothed with an osteotome (Fig. 5.16). An aluminum template is pressed tightly against the anterior aspect of the pastern bones providing an accurate reflection of the undulations of the underlying surface (Fig. 5.17).

A five-hole T-plate is contoured to conform to the anterior surfaces of the first and second phalanges and then insinuated between the extensor tendon and the underlying bone (Fig. 5.18).

Figures 5.19–5.26 deal with the application of a T-plate in the typical pastern joint arthrodesis.

Figure 5.19 shows how, with the three screws in the distal portion of the plate, the hole is prepared for the central screw by drilling a 3.2 mm hole eccentrically through the slotted hole in the T-plate.

Figures 5.20–5.26 illustrate the remainder of the surgical procedure leading to fusion of the proximal interphalangeal joint.

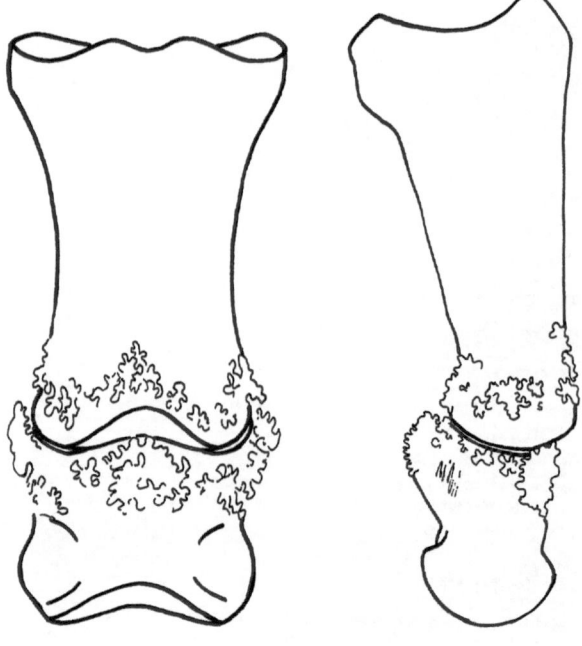

Fig. 5.12   Fig. 5.13

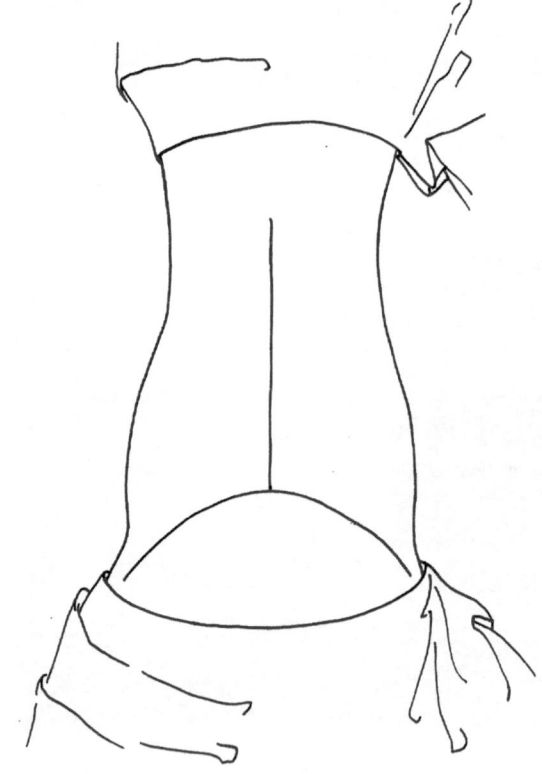

Fig. 5.14

74

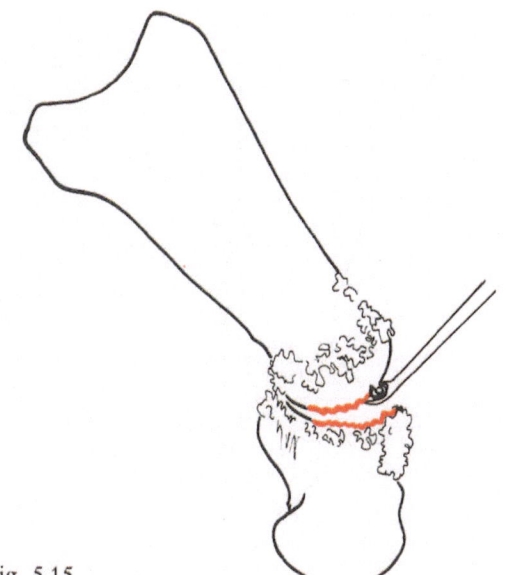

Fig. 5.15

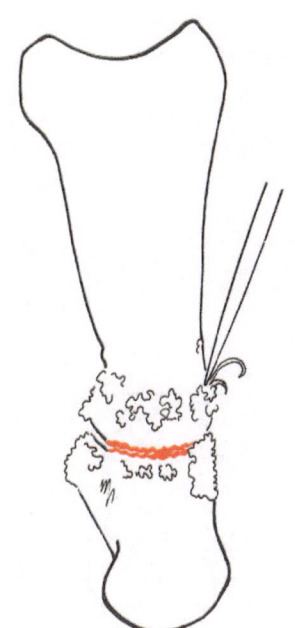

Fig. 5.16

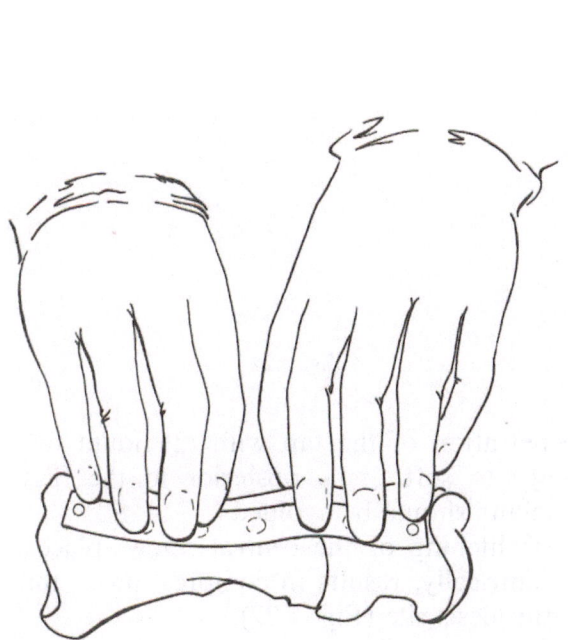

Fig. 5.17

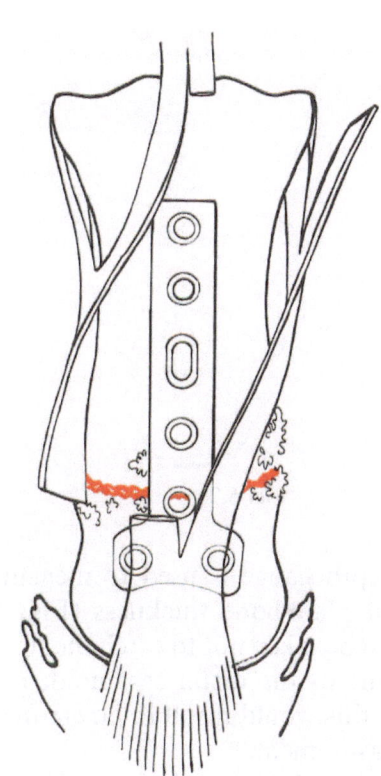

Fig. 5.18

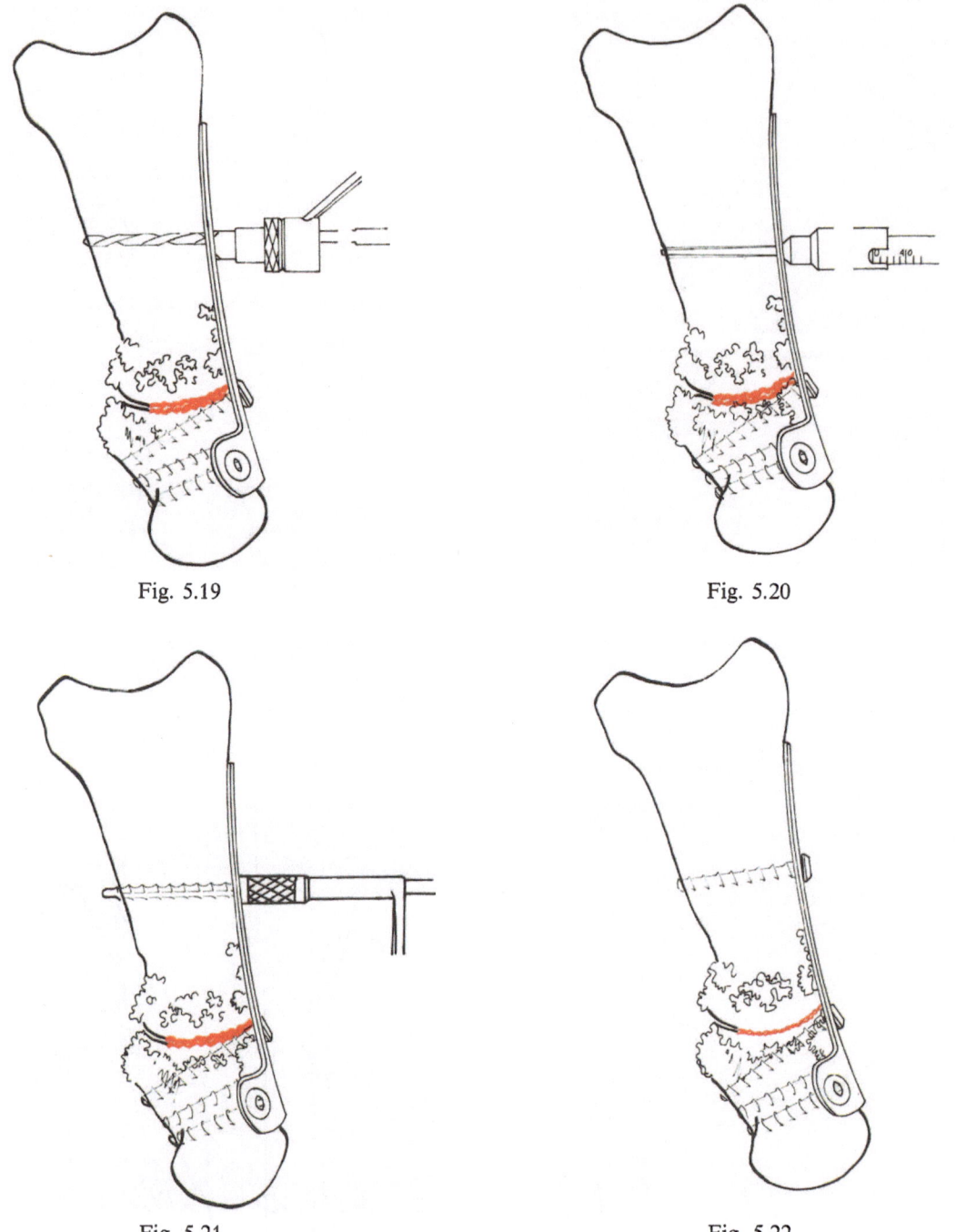

Fig. 5.19

Fig. 5.20

Fig. 5.21

Fig. 5.22

The depth gauge is used to measure the combined plate-bone thickness (Fig. 5.20). Care must be taken not to catch the tip of the instrument in the distal sesamoidean ligaments as this would result in an erroneously long measurement.

Using the 4.5 mm cortical tap, threads are cut in the 3.2 mm hole (Fig. 5.21). Excessive penetration of the tap with attendant damage to soft tissue posterior to the first phalanx should be avoided.

Tightening of the central screw, placed eccentrically, results in compression at the arthrodesis site (Fig. 5.22).

Where additional compression or reduction is required, the tension device may be

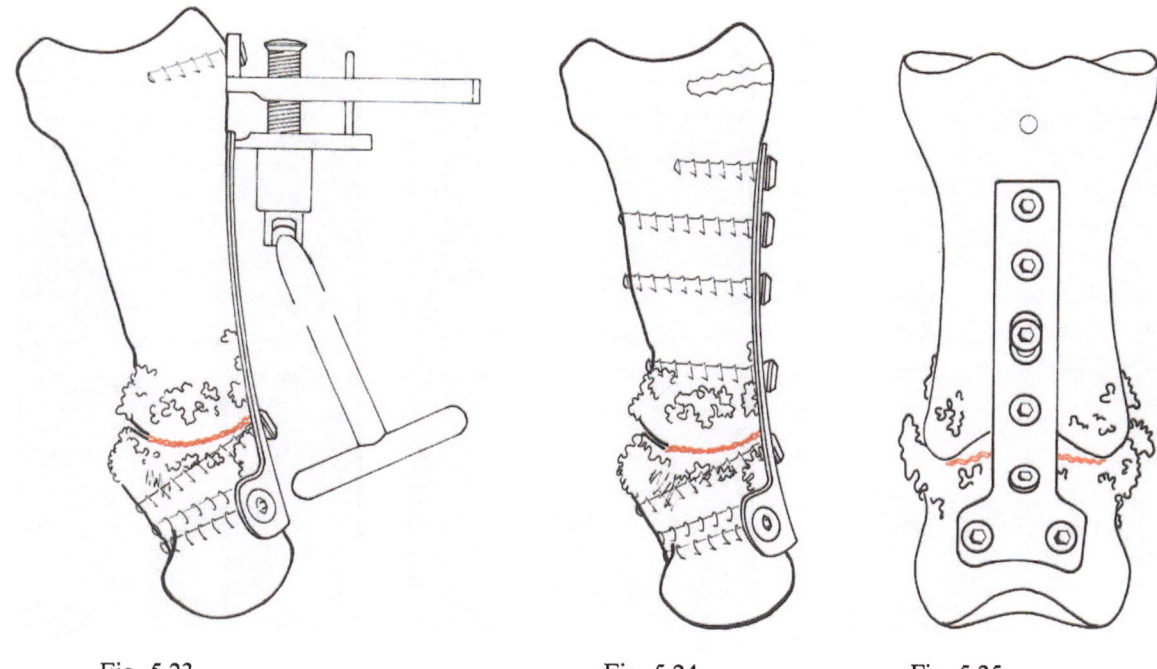

Fig. 5.23   Fig. 5.24   Fig. 5.25

attached to the proximal end of the first phalanx, as close as possible to the articular surface (Fig. 5.23). Traction upon the proximal end of the plate with this instrument effects maximal compression at the arthrodesis site.

The remaining screws are inserted in the first phalanx, and the tension device is removed (Fig. 5.24). The most proximal screw engages the anterior cortex only since the posterior cortex in this location is very thin and can contribute little to the fixation.

When properly applied, the T-plate should be accurately aligned along the longitudinal axis of the digit (Fig. 5.25).

To guard against hematoma formation at the surgical site and promote good soft-tissue healing, a suction drain is installed next to the plate prior to closure (Fig. 5.26).

Postoperatively, the operated extremity is placed in a cast from the carpus or tarsus distad. The external fixation is left in place for 6 weeks. It is then removed and replaced by a short support bandage. The horse is stall rested for a total of 12 weeks following surgery, and given positive radiographic findings, handwalking exercise is then in-

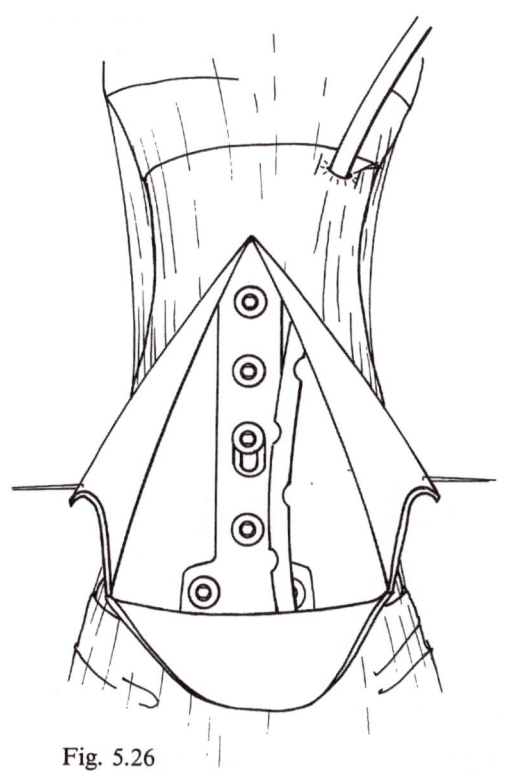

Fig. 5.26

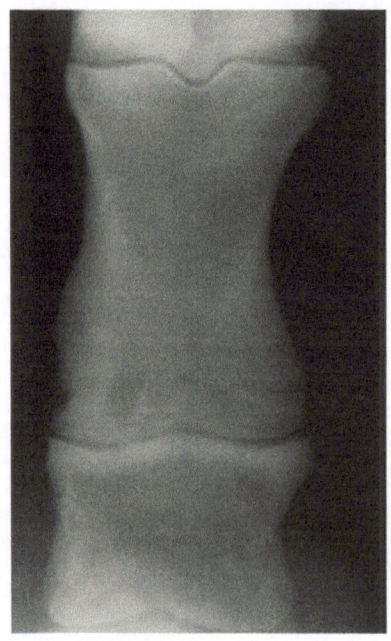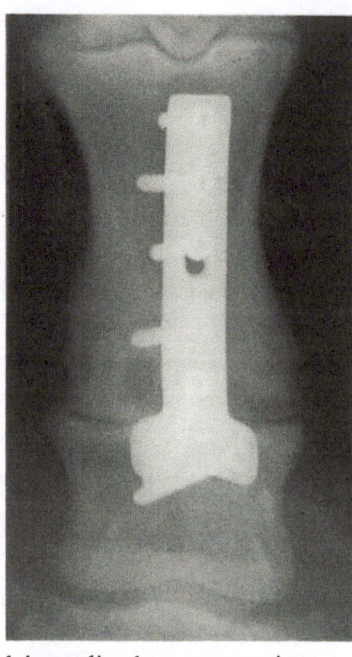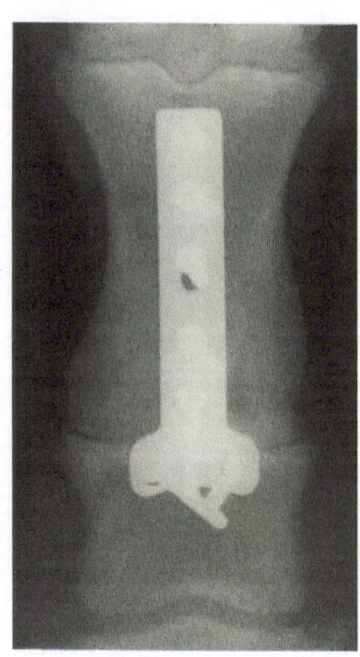

a preoperative   *b* immediately postoperative   *c* 8 weeks postoperative

Fig. 5.27 a–c

stituted. Usually, exercise at will at pasture may be permitted 16 weeks after surgery. Training is postponed a further 8 weeks and is gradually escalated according to degree of soundness. The radiographs reproduced in Fig. 5.27 a–c illustrate a typical case.

Several alternative techniques have been described for fusion of the proximal interphalangeal joint, all of which utilize some form of locally obtained cortico cancellous graft. The procedures illustrated in Figures 5.28–5.31 are two such techniques directed at

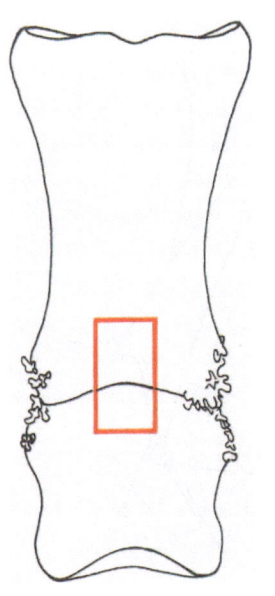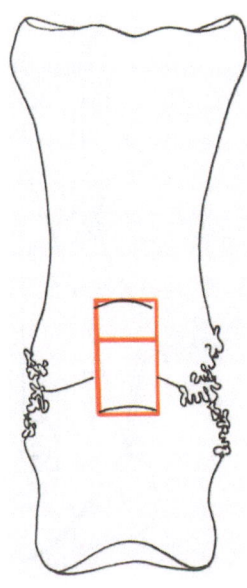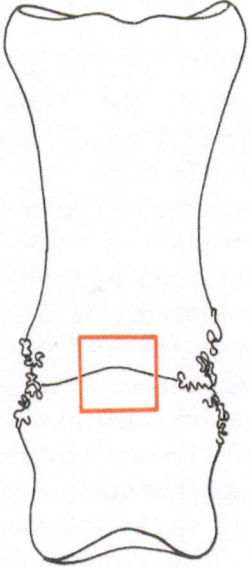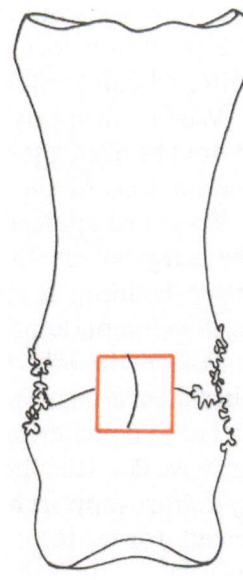

Fig. 5.28   Fig. 5.29   Fig. 5.30   Fig. 5.31

78

inducing the formation of new bone and strengthening the bridge formed across the original articular inerface.

Using an oscillating bone saw, a block of bony tissue is resected from the anterior faces of the distal aspect of the first phalanx and the proximal aspect of the second phalanx (Fig. 5.28). The proximal portion of the block is slid distally, while the second phalangeal contribution is used to fill in the resultant gap in the first phalanx (Fig. 5.29).

A second alternative is illustrated in Figures 5.30–5.31. In this variation, a square block is resected, turned through 90° and re-inserted.

Creating a greater area of contact between new cancellous surfaces should hasten un-ion, and the dove-tailing effect of the bony wedge lends to the stability of the fixation. In both cases, the application of a T-plate over the anterior surface of the phalanges is performed as previously described.

References

Schneider, JE, Carnine, BL, Guffy, MM: Arthrod-esis of the proximal interphalangeal joint in the horse: A surgical treatment for high ringbone. J. Am. Vet. Med. Assoc. *173* (1978): 1364–1369

Von Salis, B: Internal fixation in the equine: Recent advances and possible applications in private prac-tice. Proc. Am. Assoc. Equine Pract. *18* (1972): 193–218

5.2.2 Metacarpo phalangeal Joint Arthrodesis

Arthrodesis of the metacarpophalangeal joint may be indicated in chronic osteoarthritis affecting this articulation (Figs. 5.32 and 5.33). Despite sometimes extreme periarticular proliferative changes, some degrees of painful motion persist and cause lameness of varying severity. To reduce suffering, prevent breakdown of the contralateral member, and salvage the animal for breeding purposes, fusion of the joint may be considered. The technique to be described has proven effective in those cases with an intact suspensory apparatus. Where breakdown of any portion of this apparatus has taken place, additional steps, such as osteotomy of the third metacarpal bone and the first phalanx and fusion of the joint at 180° are recommended.

The *surgical approach* is through a skin incision parallel and axial to the common digital extensor tendon. The incision extends

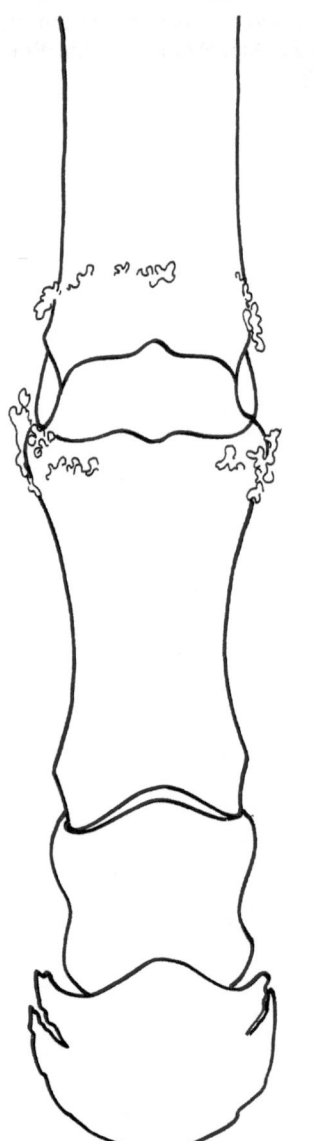

Fig. 5.32

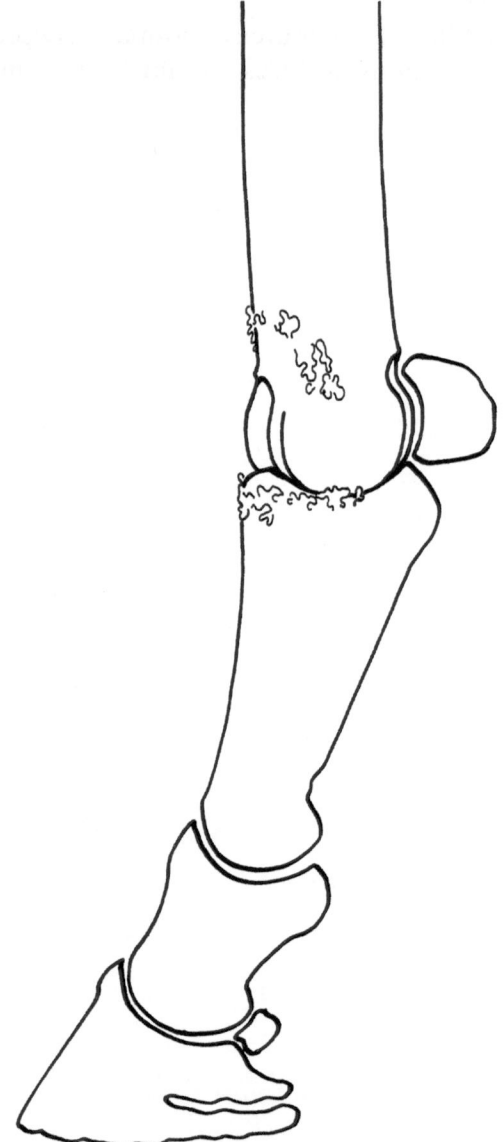

Fig. 5.33

from the proximal end of the third metacarpal bone to the level of the proximal interphalangeal joint (Fig. 5.34). Undermining the extensor tendon over this distance permits its luxation over the lateral aspect of the joint (Fig 5.35). The dorsal outpouching of the fetlock joint is then removed by a crescent-shaped incision based along the proximodorsal articular rim of the first phalanx. The distal articular surface of the third metacarpal bone is thus exposed. Partial incision of the medial and lateral collateral

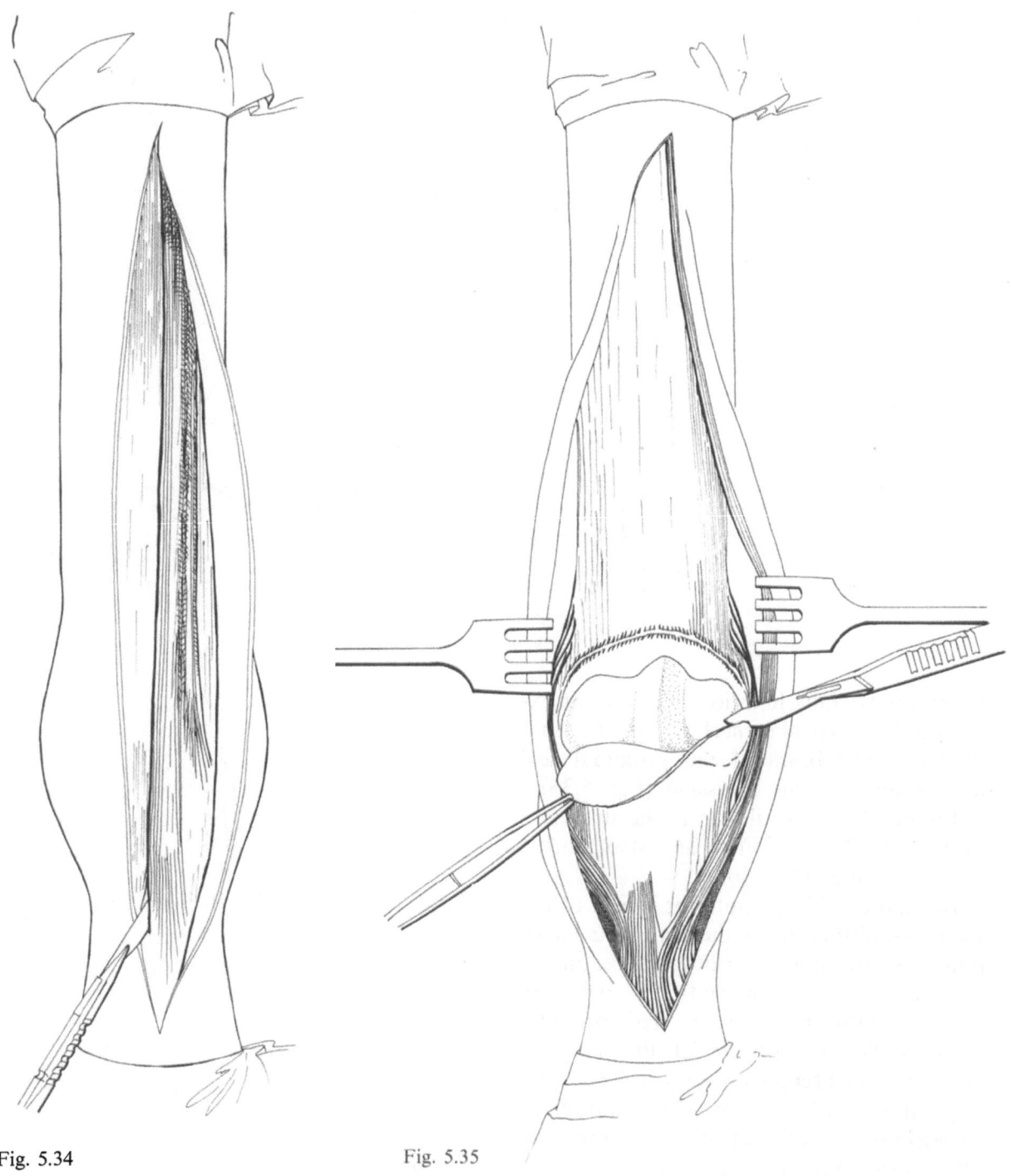

Fig. 5.34

Fig. 5.35

81

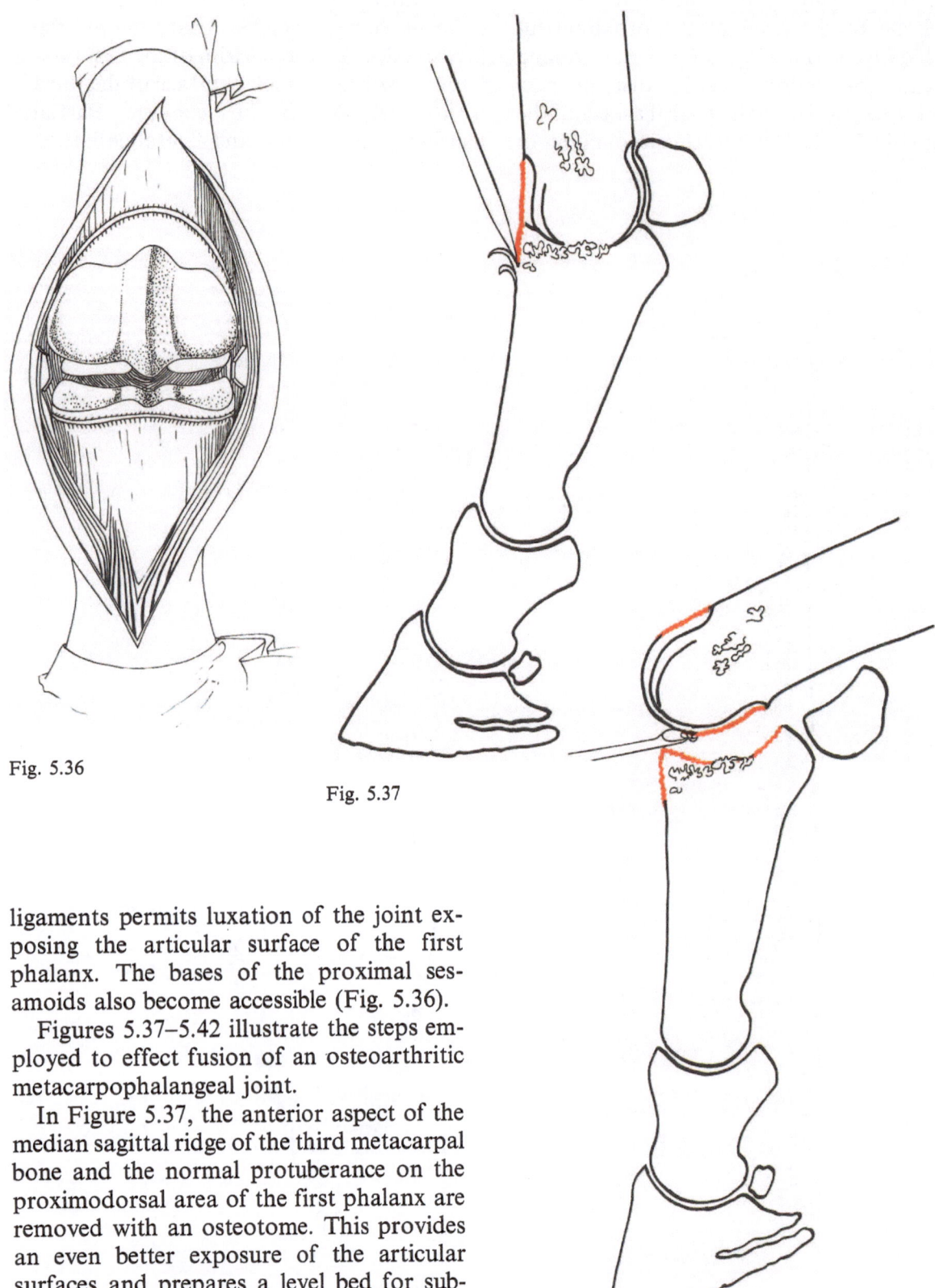

Fig. 5.36

Fig. 5.37

Fig. 5.38

ligaments permits luxation of the joint exposing the articular surface of the first
phalanx. The bases of the proximal sesamoids also become accessible (Fig. 5.36).

Figures 5.37–5.42 illustrate the steps employed to effect fusion of an osteoarthritic
metacarpophalangeal joint.

In Figure 5.37, the anterior aspect of the
median sagittal ridge of the third metacarpal
bone and the normal protuberance on the
proximodorsal area of the first phalanx are
removed with an osteotome. This provides
an even better exposure of the articular
surfaces and prepares a level bed for subsequent placement of a broad dynamic compression plate. No effort is made to remove
all periosteal proliferative changes surround-

82

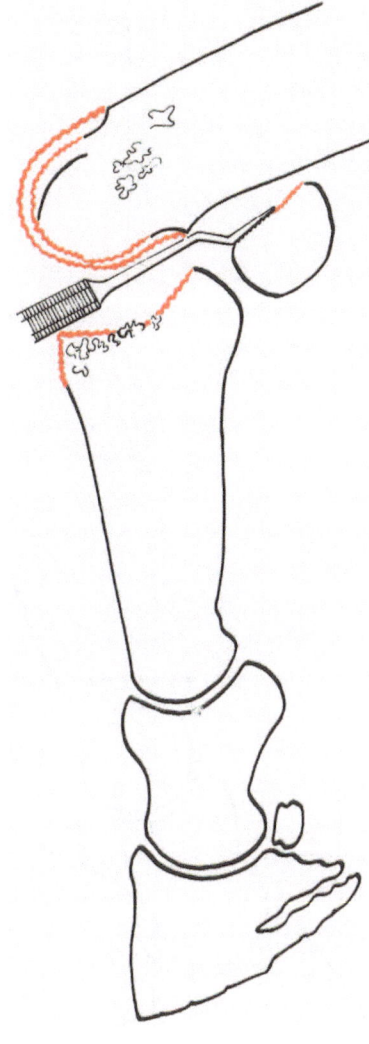

Fig. 5.39

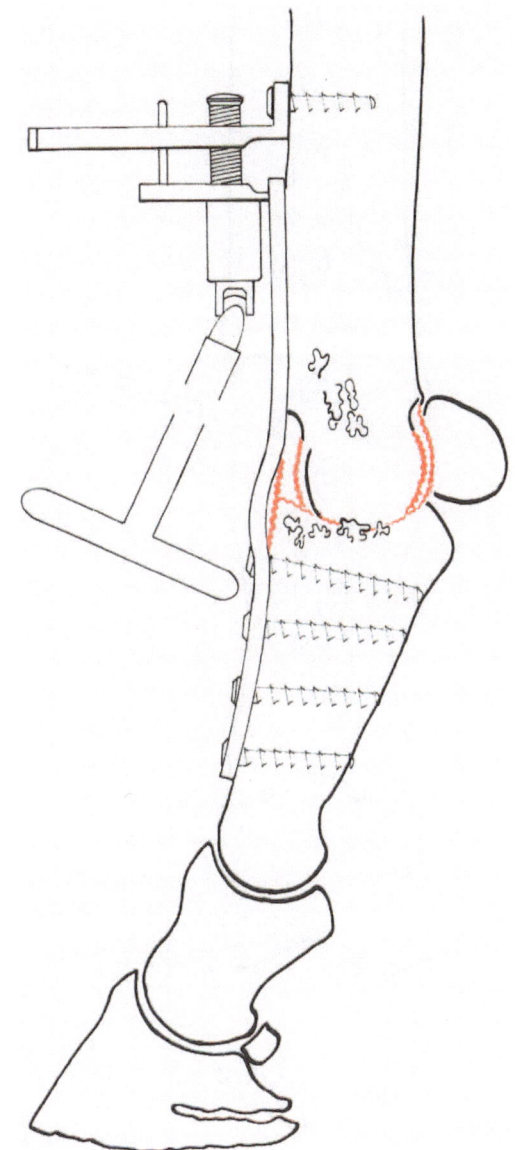

Fig. 5.40

ing the joint, as these can only contribute to later bony bridging.

The articular cartilage is removed from the joint surfaces as completely as possible (Fig. 5.38). A number of instruments may be employed for this purpose ranging from the simple curette through a mechanical burr to the ultrasonic osteotome.

A small rasp may be used to reach behind the third metacarpal bone and remove the articular cartilage from the anterior face of the proximal sesamoids (Fig. 5.39). This enhances fusion of the sesamoids to the posterior aspect of the third metacarpal bone and the additional stability conferred by the

attachments of the distal sesamoidean ligaments.

A broad eight- or nine-hole dynamic compression plate is contoured to conform to the anterior surfaces of the third metacarpal and the first phalanx (Fig. 5.40). The plate is slightly overbent at the level of the articulation in order to provide compression of the posterior region of the joint and resist the tendency toward anterior collapse of the fixation. The tension device is applied prox-

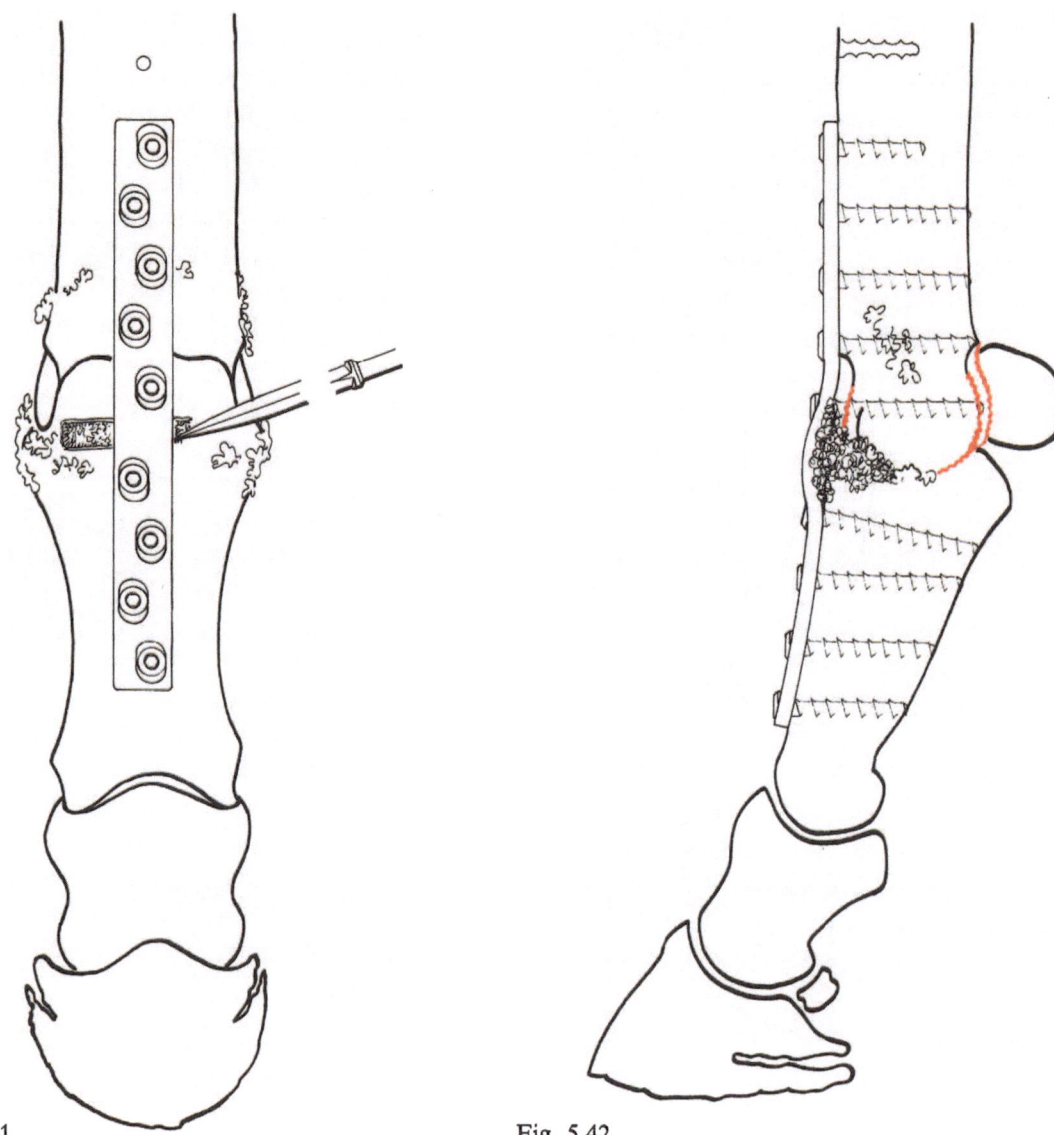

Fig. 5.41

Fig. 5.42

imally to create maximal compression at the arthrodesis site.

Following placement of the remaining proximal screws, a three-cornered bit is used to cut into the subchondral bone next to the plate (Fig. 5.41).

Cancellous bone is packed into the arthrodesis site under and around the plate to accelerate osteogenesis and promote fusion (Fig. 5.42).

Postoperatively, a suction drain is placed beneath the extensor tendons, which are replaced over the plate, and the operated extremity is placed in a cast from the carpus distad. The cast is reset at 6 weeks and can usually be removed at 12 weeks postoperatively. While the external fixation is in place, the horse is stall rested. Thereafter, handwalking exercise for gradually increasing periods of time is instituted. Usually, the animal may begin to exercise at will at pasture approximately 20 weeks after surgery. With time, bone grows up to and around the plate, which need not be removed. The radiographs in Fig. 5.43 a-d document the progress of a typical case.

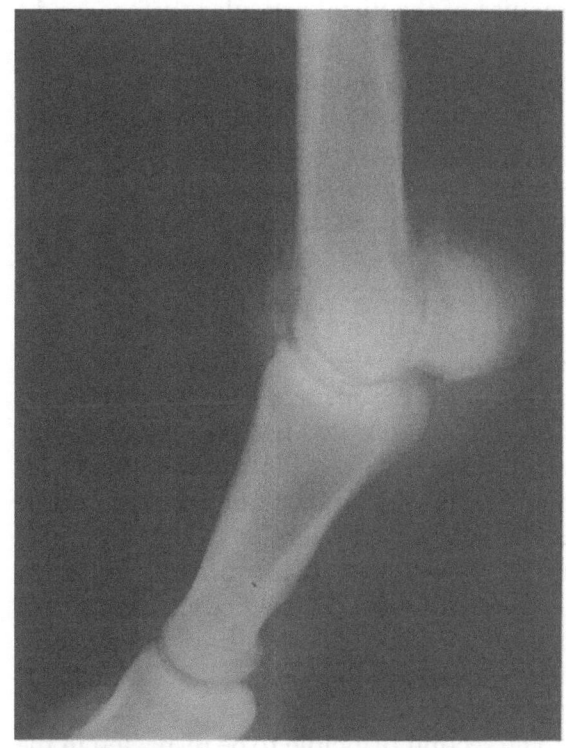

a preoperative

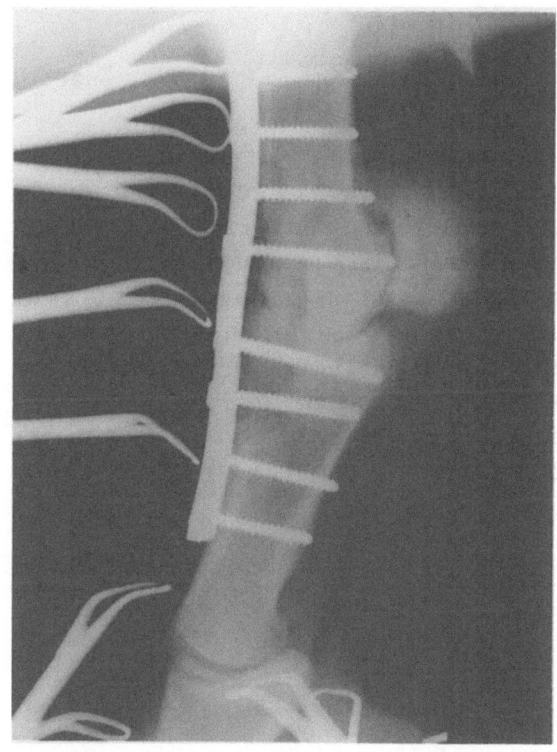

b immediately postoperative

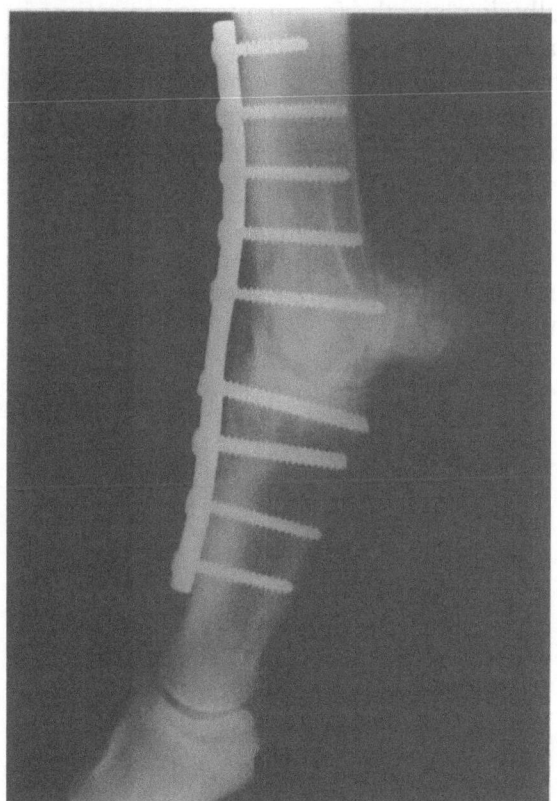

c 12 weeks postoperative
Fig. 5.43 a–d

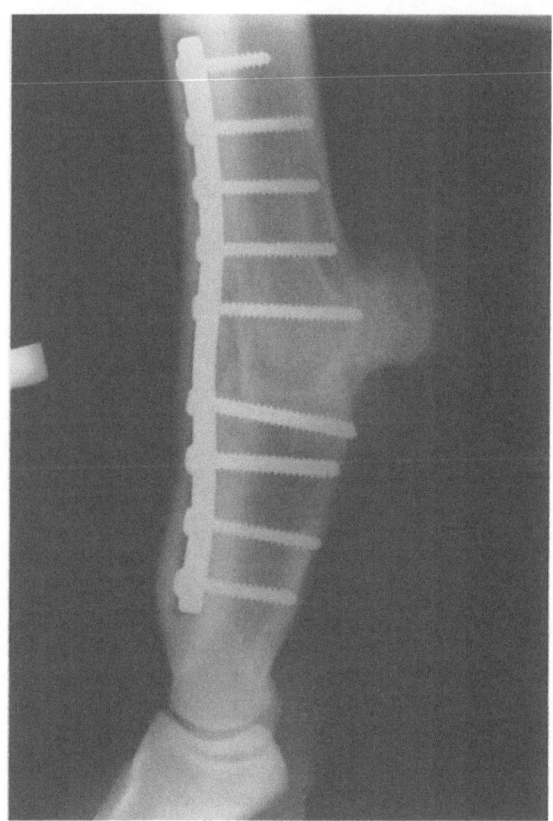

d 52 weeks postoperative

5.3 Comminuted Fractures of the First Phalanx

Comminuted fractures of the first phalanx are common racehorse injuries and probably begin during fast-gaited exercise as simple sagittal or frontal fractures of the bone that rapidly proliferate as the animal continues to run and cannot be stopped in time to prevent further damage. Though these fractures are extremely variable in their exact configurations, they usually consist of a cruciate combination of sagittal and frontal fractures of the proximal articular surface, a sagittal fracture of the distal articular surface, and a variable amount of fragmentation of the midportion of the bone (Fig. 5.44).

Associated with these fractures are meaningful soft-tissue injuries. Subperiosteal hemorrhage and hemorrhage into the soft tissues surrounding the fetlock joint and the suspensory apparatus are often severe. Further hemorrhaging into the digital sheath and the metacarpophalangeal joint itself is also common.

One of the first principles important in the repair of comminuted fractures is to provide adequate exposure. A double flap incision is made in the skin on the anterior aspect of the fetlock and pastern similar to that described for arthrodesis of the proximal interphalangeal joint (Fig. 5.14). A Z-incision in the extensor tendon allows it to be reflected laterally and medially exposing the underlying bone.

The second principle to be respected in the repair of comminuted fractures is to carefully displace the fragments one at a time in an effort to gain a better understanding of their relationships, but not to displace them so far as to create further, seemingly insurmountable instability. Once the surgeon has gained an understanding of at least one portion of the fracture, that particular portion should be reduced and secured. This meaningfully simplifies dealing with the remaining pieces.

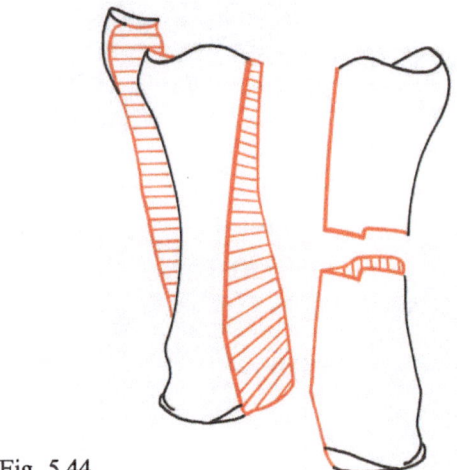

Fig. 5.44

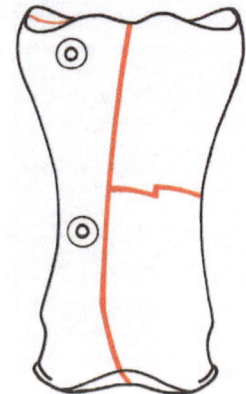

Fig. 5.45

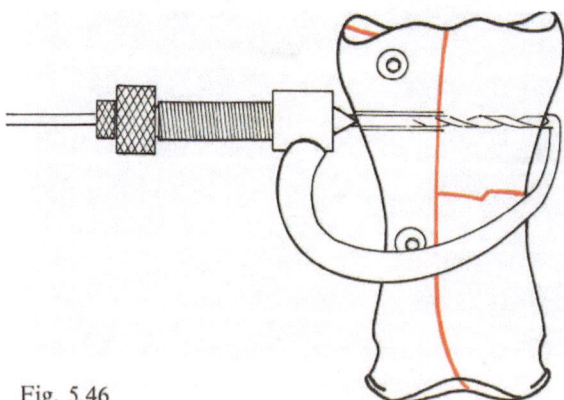

Fig. 5.46

Figure 5.45 shows lag screws placed from anterior to posterior bridging the frontal fracture on the lateral aspect of the proximal end of the first phalanx. A C-clamp is then placed as a reduction instrument, and a drill guide allowing gliding and pilot holes to be prepared to accept a screw bridging the proximal mid sagittal fracture (Fig. 5.46).

The pilot hole is tapped through the C-clamp as described in Chapter 4, following which a second lag screw is placed parallel to the first, reducing three original fragments to only one.

The C-clamp is again employed to reduce the distal sagittal fracture and to act as a drill guide for the preparation of a hole to accept the distal most lag screw, which places the sagittal fracture of the distal articular surface under compression (Fig. 5.47).

With these four screws in place the only instability remaining is that due to the trans-verse fracture through the medial portion of the bone. This fracture may be bridged by a T-plate, which after careful contouring, is placed across the fracture plane as shown in Figures 5.48 and 5.49. Such a plate is sometimes referred to as a neutralization plate since it acts not only to stabilize a portion of the fracture but also to maintain length and protect the interfragmentary screws against shear forces.

Soft-tissue closure is routine comprising careful adaptation of the extensor tendon and fascial flaps, suction drainage (Fig. 5.26), subcuticular suturing, and closure of the skin. Since the reconstruction of such comminuted fractures does not constitute a fixation capable of resisting the forces of unrestricted weight bearing, a fiberglass cast is applied at the conclusion of surgery and maintained over a period of six to twelve weeks.

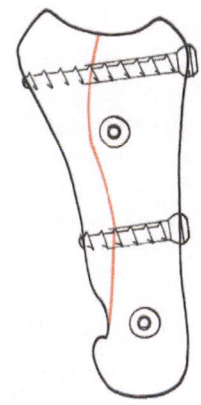

Fig. 5.47

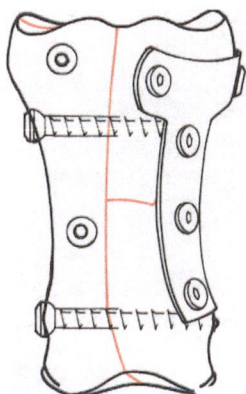

Fig. 5.48

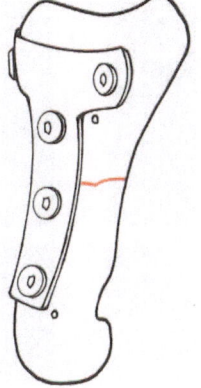

Fig. 5.49

87

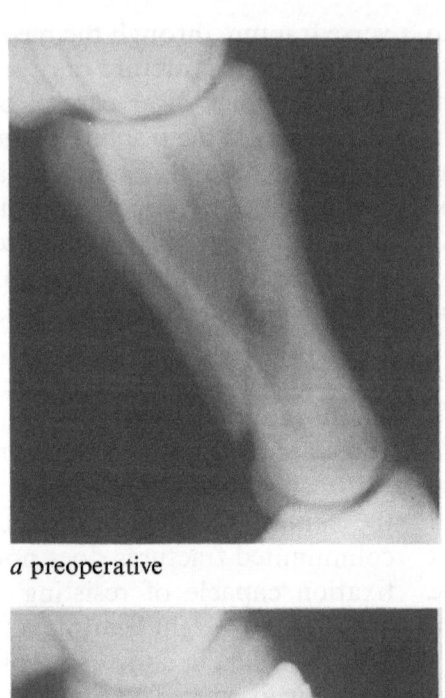

a preoperative

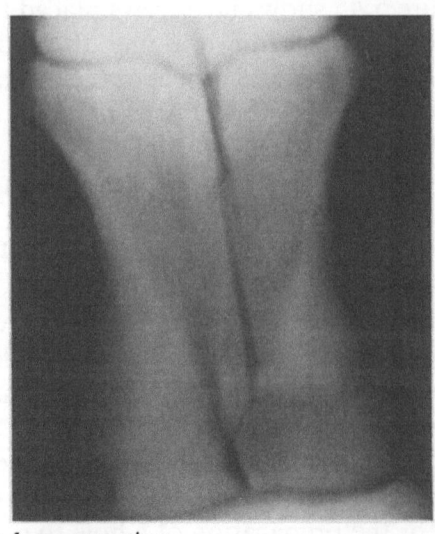

b preoperative

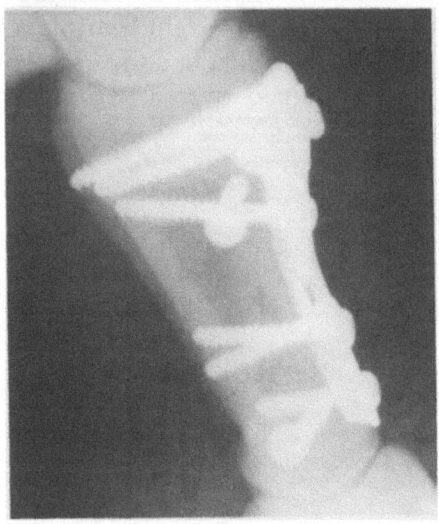

c immediately postoperative

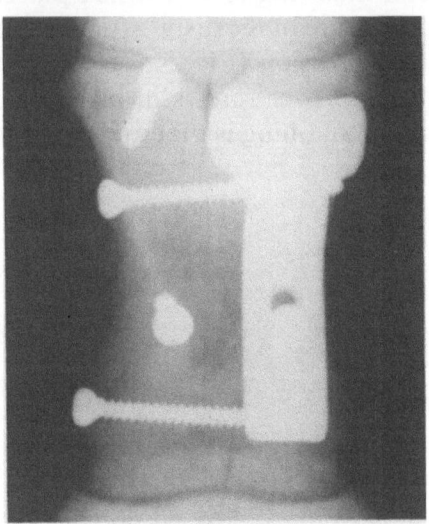

d immediately postoperative

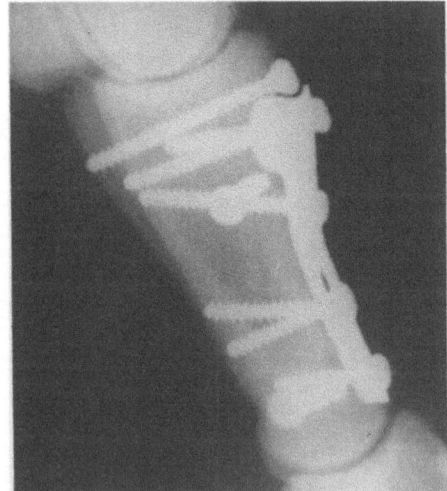

e 6 weeks postoperative
Fig. 5.50 a–f

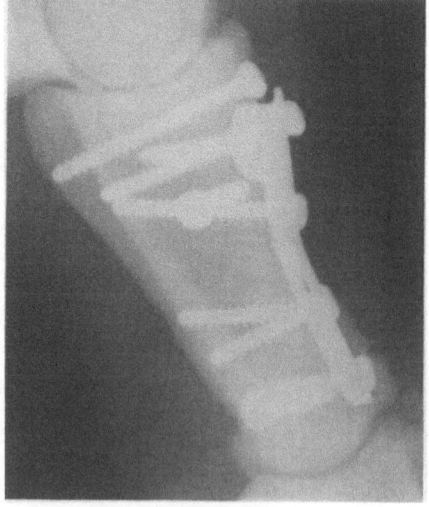

f 12 weeks postoperative

88

The radiographs reproduced in Fig. 5.50a–f document the progress of a typical case. The osteoarthritic changes seen developing in the proximal interphalangeal joint are due partially to the damage done to the articular surface by the fracture, and partially to the instability of this joint secondary to traumatic disruption of the oblique sesamoidean ligaments. This subluxation can sometimes be severe and require a secondary arthrodesis of the proximal interphalangeal joint. The frequency of the occurrence of this lesion as a long term complication has led us in more recent cases to the performance of an arthrodesis at the time of the initial fracture repair.

Following successful repair, afflicted horses may be used as breeding animals for many years and are able to exercise at pasture without pain. As the normal axis of the limb is maintained, secondary degenerative changes and angular deformities at other joints of the injured extremity are minimized.

Reference

Bowman, KF, Fackelman, GE: The management of comminuted fractures in the horse. Compend. vet. cont. educ. *2* (1980): 98–102

Chapter 6. Growth Plate Retardation

6.1 Distal Radius

Angular limb deformity due to metaphyseal dysplasia (Fig. 6.1) is a common malady afflicting the distal radius in the young growing foal. The deformity responds well to growth plate retardation. The affected animal shows an abnormal curvature of the radius proximal to the growth plate causing the limb distal to that point to deviate laterally. The lateral aspect of the distal radius is strongly concave or "dished," although radiographically, the true epiphysis of the bone will show the normal rectangular configuration. In making the diagnosis, care should be taken to differentiate the condition from the various other abnormalities of the carpus that can result in similar clinical appearances. A similar condition may affect the distal tibia and can be treated by essentially the same surgical procedure.

The *surgical approach* is through an approximately 50 mm skin incision from a point proximal to the medial radial epicondyle to the level of the radiocarpal joint. A 20 gauge hypodermic needle may be used to mark the location and plane of the growth plate (Fig. 6.2).

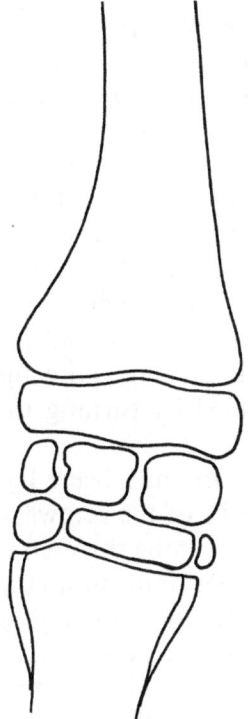

Fig. 6.1

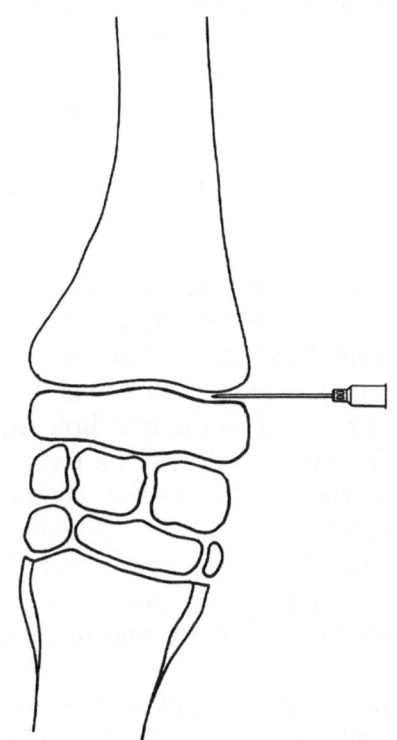

Fig. 6.2

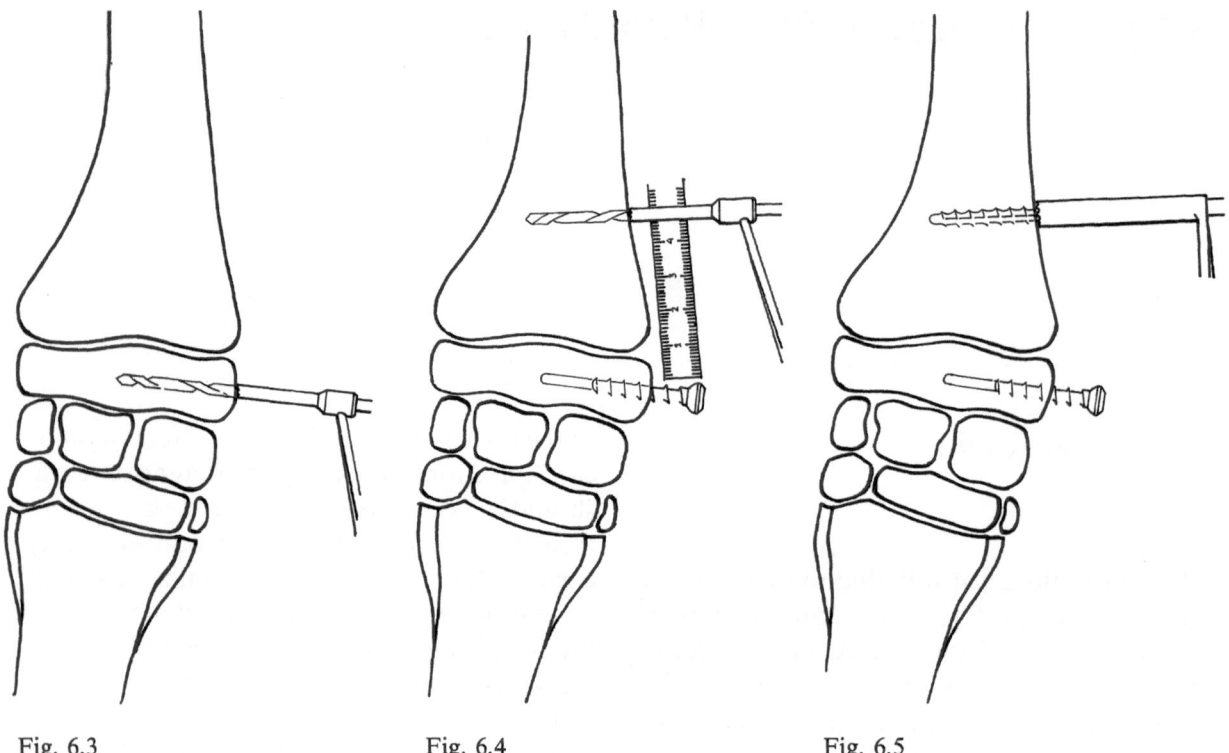

Fig. 6.3   Fig. 6.4   Fig. 6.5

Figures 6.3–6.14 illustrate a technique of growth plate retardation proven effective in correcting this class of deformity.

Figure 6.3 shows how, by means of the 3.2 mm drill bit inserted through the 3.5 mm tap sleeve, a 3.2 mm hole is prepared on the medial aspect of the distal radius centered in the epiphysis and parallel to the growth plate and hence also parallel to the articular surface. The hole is carried to a depth of 34–36 mm.

A regular 4.5 mm cortical bone screw is inserted in self-tapping fashion to ensure a tight hold in the soft bone of the epiphysis (Fig. 6.4). A second 3.2 mm hole is drilled 50 mm proximal to the first hole, again using the 3.5 mm tap sleeve as a tissue protector. Only the medial radial cortex need be penetrated.

Using the 4.5 mm cortical tap through the 4.5 mm tap sleeve, threads are cut in the denser bone of the radial metaphysis (Fig. 6.5).

The second 4.5 mm cortical bone screw is inserted in the medial distal radial metaphysis (Fig. 6.6). Neither screw is tightened, so that both protrude from the surrounding tissues. Alternatively, in very young foals, the surgeon might opt to use cancellous screws and their corresponding tap and tap sleeve.

A loop of 1.2 mm cerclage wire, approximately 60 mm in diameter, is prepared by passing the free end of the wire through the eye in the other end (Fig. 6.7). The loop is then twisted into a figure-of-eight.

The figure-of-eight of cerclage wire is fitted to the heads of the screws so that the eye in the wire is in the deeper throw of the loop (Fig. 6.8). The free end of the wire is engaged by the cerclage wire tightener and tension is created by turning the handle of the instrument.

When the wire has been lightly tensed against the necks of the screws, the cerclage wire tightener is swung through 90°, creating a hook-in-eye configuration (Fig. 6.9).

With the cerclage wire tightener still in place, the screws are tightened (Fig. 6.10). Additional tension is thereby brought about in the wire as it slides along the inclined plane

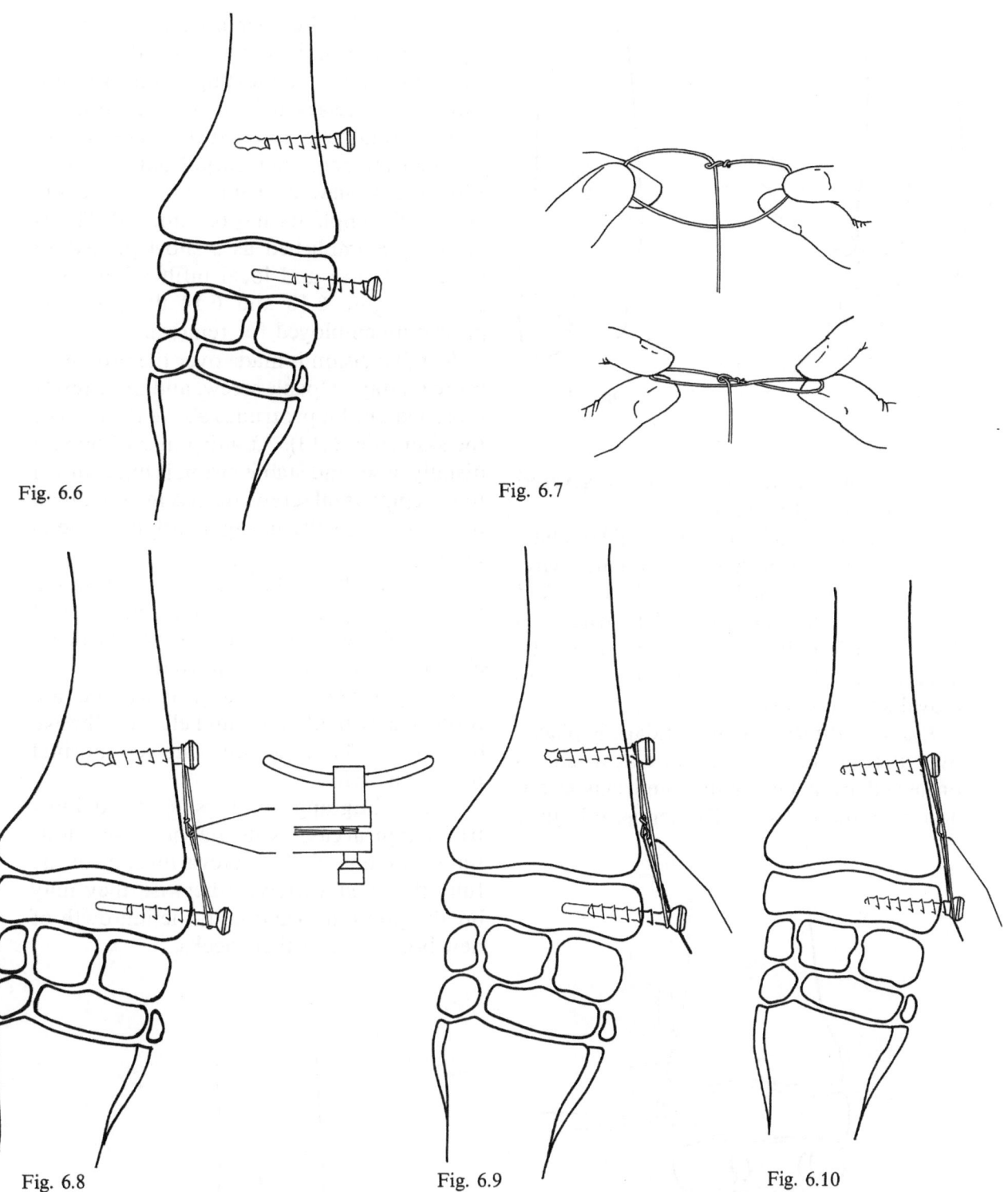

Fig. 6.6

Fig. 6.7

Fig. 6.8

Fig. 6.9

Fig. 6.10

of the underside of the spherical screw heads. Neither screw should be maximally tightened as the wire might slip off over the heads. The distal screw will require less tightening

due to the interposition of the medial collateral ligament.

After turning the handle of the cerclage wire tightener in the direction of loosening,

93

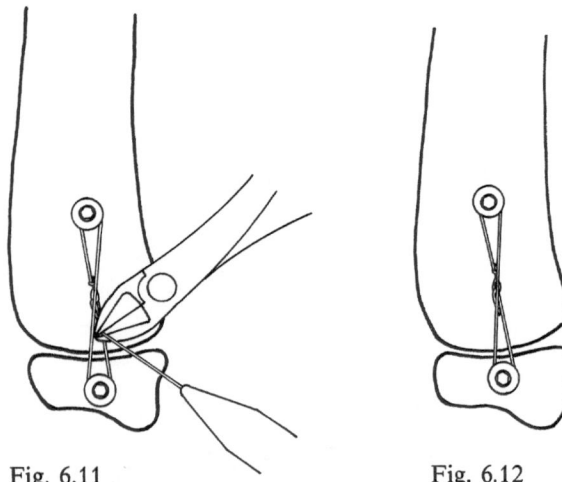

Fig. 6.11   Fig. 6.12

the 1–2 mm cerclage wire may be severed near the hook (Fig. 6.11).

The finished configuration should be characterized by well-placed screws, tense wire, and a neatly formed hook-in-eye tucked under the superficial throw of the wire loop (Fig. 6.12). The hook in the wire should be directed distally to provide for easier removal subsequently.

Postoperatively, a stent bandage is placed over the wound, and the operative site is protected by a light gauze and elastic adhesive bandage. The foal's exercise is limited until the limbs show significant straightening, so that secondary changes in the hooves and soft-tissue supporting elements are avoided. Exercise can be increased toward a more normal level as correction continues.

When the radiometacarpal axis becomes 180° when viewed from in front of the animal, the implants may be removed. This is usually accomplished as a short procedure under sedation and local infiltration anesthesia. Figure 6.13 and 6.14 illustrate the procedure employed for removal.

A stab incision is made over the proximal, more readily palpable screw, and the screw is loosened until it protrudes above the level of the skin (Fig. 6.13). At a distance of 50 mm distally, a second stab incision is made down to the epiphyseal screw. Both screws are then removed using the hexagonal-tipped screwdriver.

A curved hemostatic forceps is inserted through the proximal incision and hooked beneath the wire loop (Fig. 6.14). With an abrupt tug, the wire is removed.

Postoperatively, the surgical wounds are protected by light gauze and elastic adhesive bandages. The foals are allowed normal pasture activity.

The radiographs in Figs. 6.15a–d illustrate a typical case. Note that here cancellous screws were used. The screws must be of the fully-threaded variety, otherwise they may break upon removal due to the ingrowth of new bone around their necks.

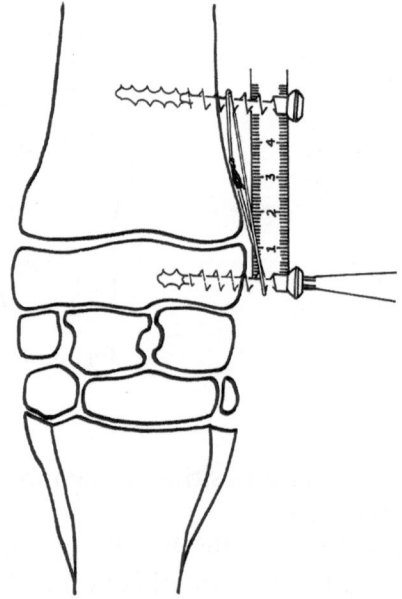

Fig. 6.13

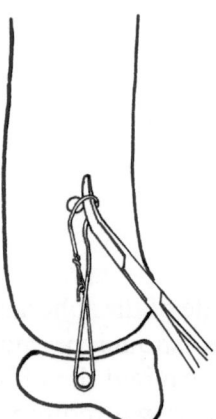

Fig. 6.14

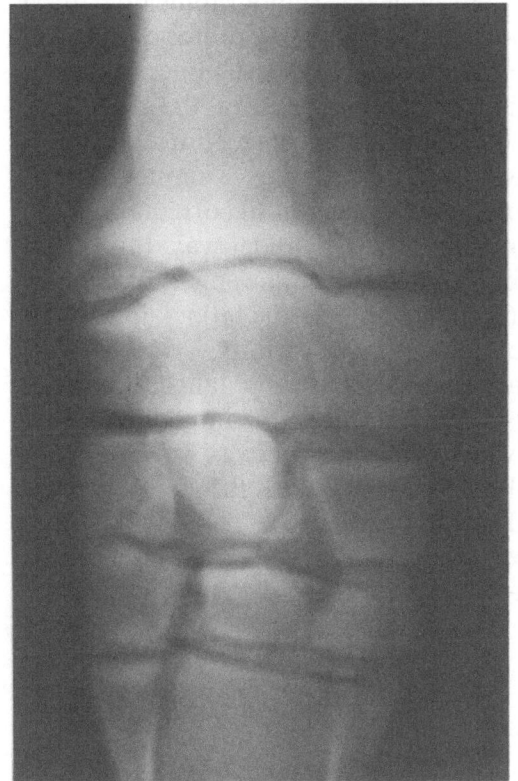

a preoperative

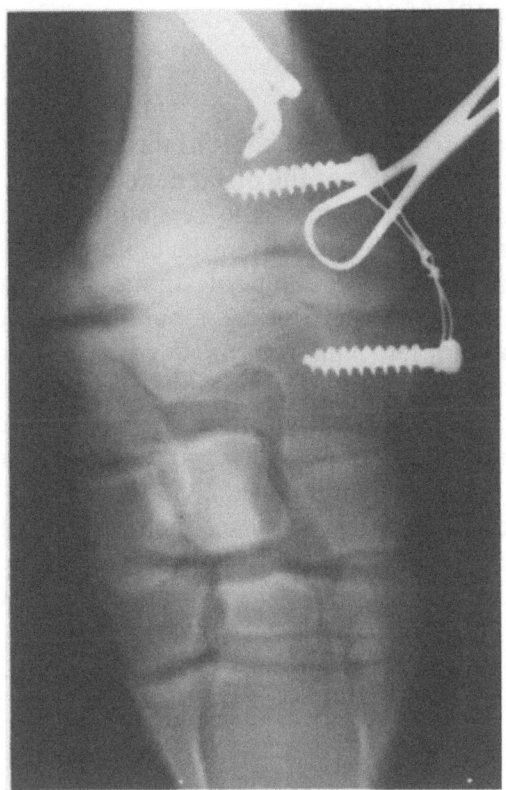

b immediately postoperative

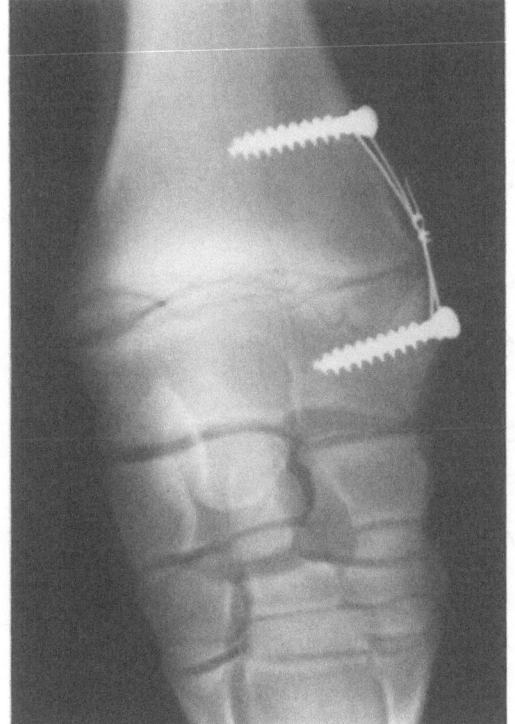

c 9 weeks postoperative

Fig. 6.15   a–d

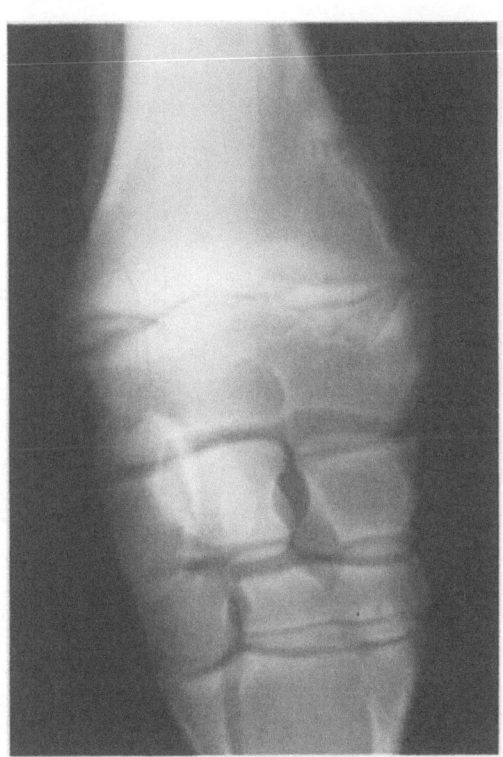

d 9 weeks postoperative following implant removal

95

6.2 Distal Metacarpus and Metatarsus

Deviations from a normal axis in the region of the growth plates of the distal metacarpal or metatarsal bones are usually secondary to direct trauma. Fibrosis within the collateral ligament and surrounding soft tissues, including the periosteum of the area, bridges the growth plate and retards the rate of proliferation on the traumatized side. Growth continues at a normal rate on the other side of the plate causing the limb to deviate *toward* the injured side. Commonly, the true epiphysis becomes secondarily deformed, exaggerating the deformity (Fig. 6.16).

If there appears, radiographically, to be any potential for further proliferation at the injured aspect of the growth plate, surgically bridging the convex side of the deformity (Fig. 6.17) may effect correction.

Postoperatively, exercise is limited to stall rest and handwalking until correction of the axis of the limb is well under way. It is hoped thereby to avert the development of secondary arthritic change in the fetlock joints and concomitant hoof deformity.

When the metacarpophalangeal axis becomes 180° (Fig. 6.18), the implants may be removed as described above.

Following correction, the foals are allowed normal exercise.

The radiographs reproduced in Figures 6.19a–c illustrate a typical case.

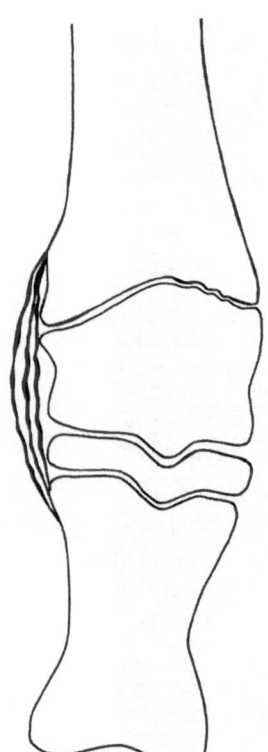

Fig. 6.16

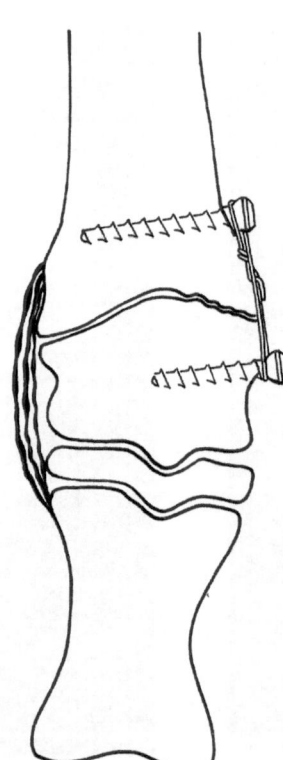

Fig. 6.17

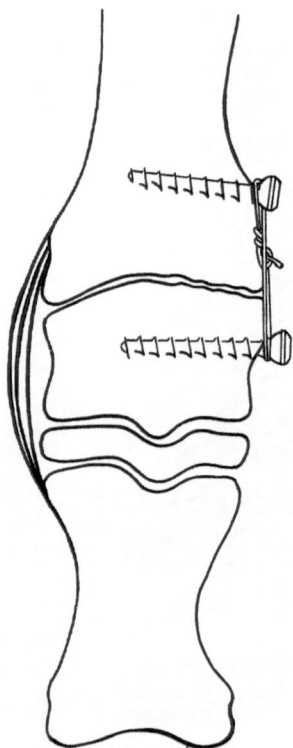

Fig. 6.18

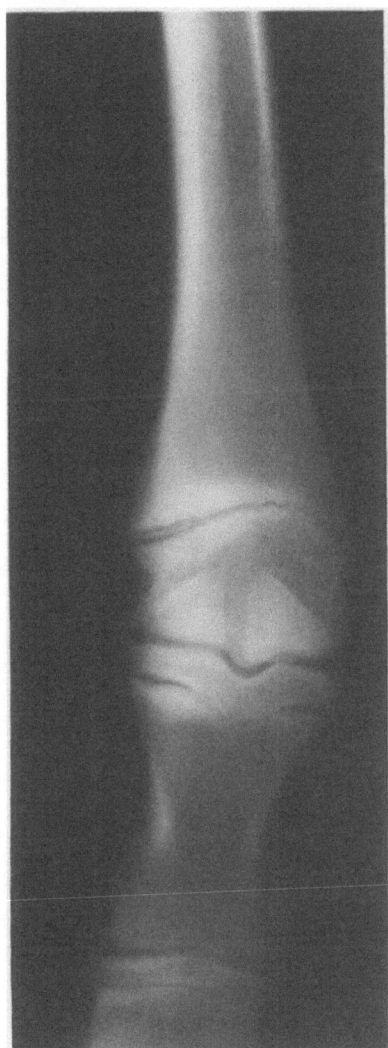 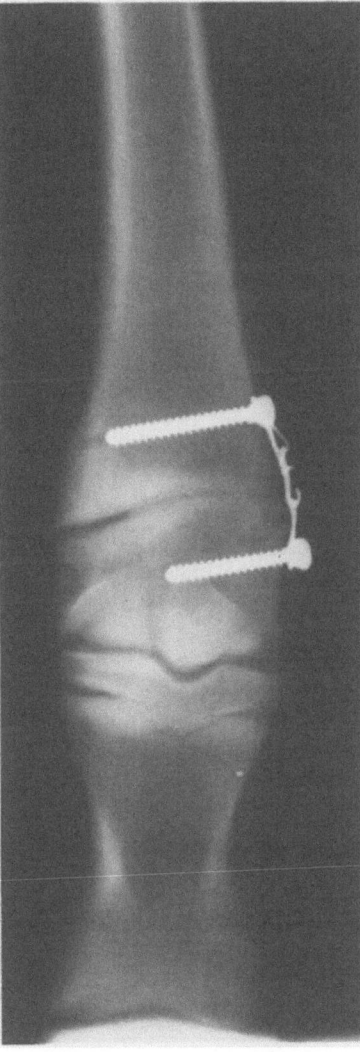 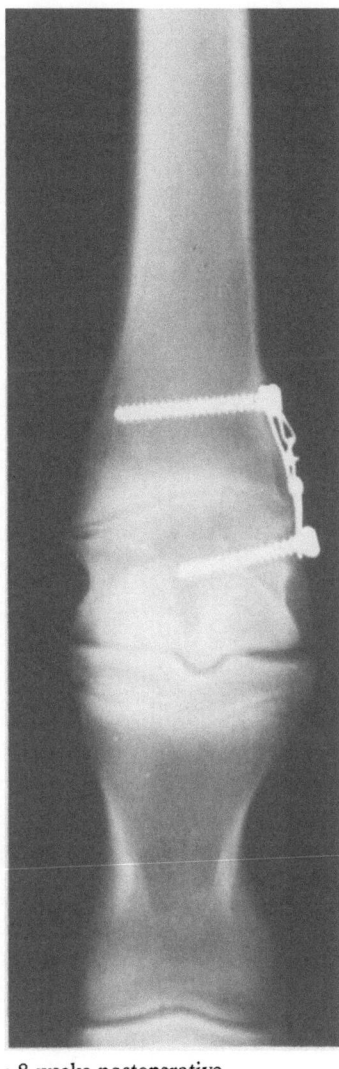

a preoperative   *b* immediately postoperative   *c* 8 weeks postoperative

Fig. 6.19 a–c

References

Auer, J, Martens, R: Angular limb deformities in young foals. Proc. Amer. Assoc. Equine Pract. *26* (1980): 89–96

Fackelman, GE, Reid, CF, Leitch, M, Cimprich, R: Angular limb deformities in foals. Proc. Am. Assoc. Equine Pract. *21* (1975): 161–166

Fretz, PB, Turner, AS, Pharr, J: Retrospective comparison of two surgical techniques for correction of angular deformities in foals. J. Am. Vet. Med. Assoc. *172* (1975): 281–286

Leitch, M: Angular limb deformities arising at the carpal region in foals. Compend. vet. cont. educ. *1* (1979): 39–43

Chapter 7. Bone Grafting

Bone healing under conditions of stable internal fixation has frequently been referred to as a race between the body's ability to proliferate new osseous tissue and the implant's ability to withstand and counteract the stresses to which it is subjected. Any technique or procedure that serves to tip the balance in favor of the bone will enhance a favorable outcome of the case under consideraction.

The placement of cancellous bone in or around the site of a fracture, osteotomy, pseudoarthrosis, or arthrodesis has been observed to accelerate bony union. The mechanism by which this occurs is still the subject of active debate and research as it appears that elements of the graft and elements of the surrounding recipient tissues both participate in the formation of new bone. Which elements are most important in any given instance may be related to histocompatibility, site of implantation, or time since grafting.

The material most commonly employed in grafting is fresh autologous cancellous bone. The sites from which this bone is harvested include the tuber coxae, the proximal tibia, the sternum, or the ribs. Since the first-stated location is the one most frequently employed, the surgery involved in obtaining cancellous bone from that site will be described. Most surgeons opt to harvest grafts from the tuber coxae unless positioning of the patient precludes a convenient approach.

The approach described here represents a modification of those previously performed and permits the extraction of a maximal amount of material through a minimal exposure.

With the patient in lateral recumbency the area over the iliac wing is clipped, disinfected and draped preparatory to aseptic surgery. A semilunar skin incision is made creating a dorsally based flap over the ventral most portion of the tuber coxae (Fig. 7.1).

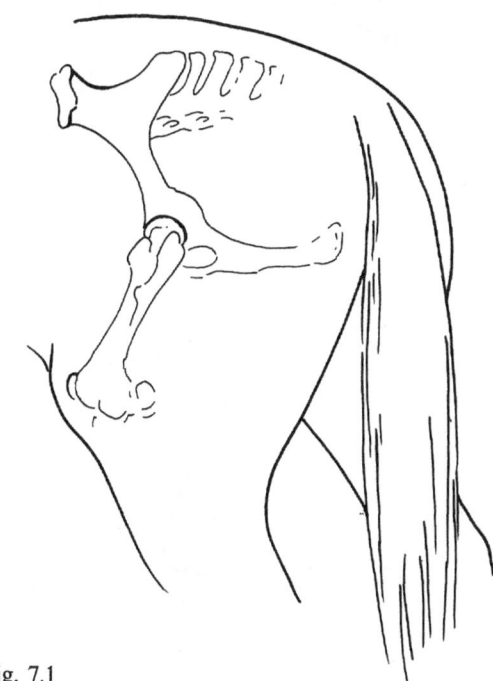

Fig. 7.1

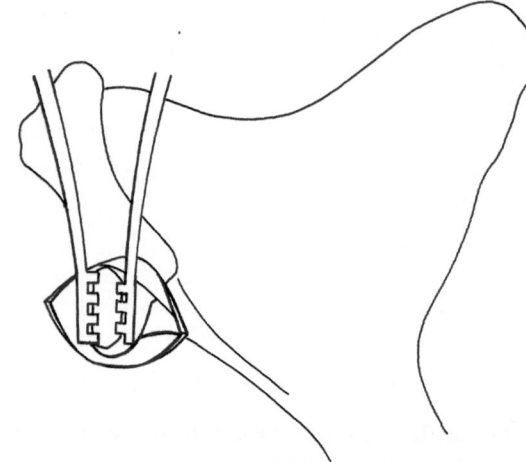

Fig. 7.2

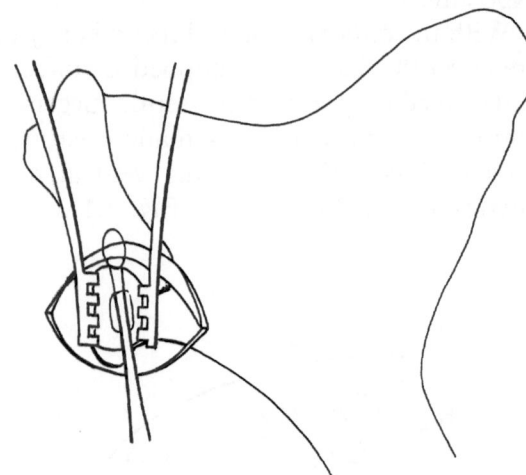

Fig. 7.4

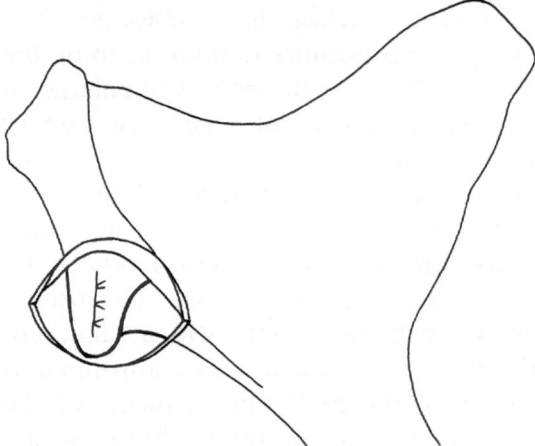

Fig. 7.5

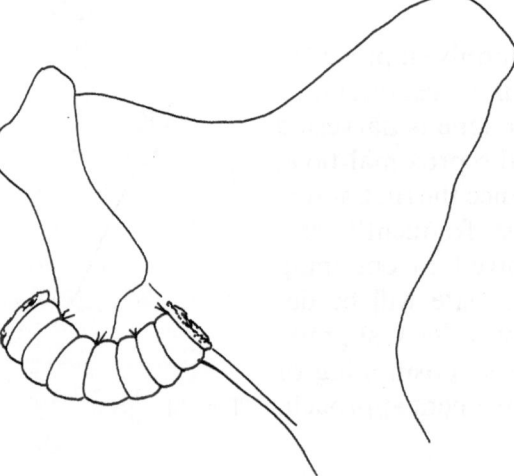

Fig. 7.6

A short straight incision is made through the gluteal and internal oblique fascia until bone is encountered (Fig. 7.2).

The cortical bone is resected using a gouge, exposing the underlying red, fatty medullary tissues (Fig. 7.3).

Using a curette directed axially, dorsally and somewhat anteriorly, cancellous bone from the interior of the entire tuber coxae and part of the wing of the ilium may be removed through a relatively small opening (Fig. 7.4).

The deep fascia and periosteal tissues are sutured over the defect (Fig. 7.5). Following subcuticular and skin suturing, a stent bandage is placed to protect the wound (Fig. 7.6).

By proceeding in this fashion, one of the major disadvantages of obtaining grafts from the hip, wound dehiscence and subsequent osteomyelitis, can be minimized. The cancellous grafts significantly expedite healing and are especially valuable in badly comminuted fractures, where they may be used to replace missing or devitalized cortical segments.

Addressing the more general disadvantage of autologous bone grafting: the necessity of a second piece of surgery on an already traumatized patient; recent work has demonstrated the practicality of banking homologous bone for future use. Should clinical use verify the apparently favorable preliminary findings, the technique might assume a vital role in the treatment of fractures in large animals.

References

Fackelman, GE, von Rechenberg, B: Decalcified bone grafts in the horse. Am. J. Vet. Res. *42* (1981): 943–948

Slocum, B, Chalman, JA: Cancellous bone grafts from the wing of the equine ilium – a surgical approach. Arch. Am. Coll. Vet. Surg. *4* (1975): 39–45

General References

Hickman, J, Walker, RG: An Atlas of Veterinary Surgery. JB Lippincott Co., Philadelphia-Toronto 1973

Leonard, EP: Orthopedic Surgery of the Dog and Cat. WB Saunders Co., Philadelphia-London-Toronto 1971

Matter, P, Rittmann, W: The Open Fracture. Hans Huber, Bern 1978

Milne, DW, Turner, AS: An Atlas of Surgical Approaches to the Bones of the Horse. WB Saunders Co., Philadelphia-London-Toronto 1979

Müller, ME, Allgöwer, M, Schneider, R, Willenegger, H: Manual of Osteosynthesis. Springer-Verlag, Berlin-Heidelberg-New York 1977

Pauwels, F: Biomechanics of the Locomotor Apparatus. Springer-Verlag, Berlin-Heidelberg-New York 1980

Peacock, EE, van Winkle, W: Wound Repair. WB Saunders Co., Philadelphia-London-Toronto 1976

Piermattei, DL, Greeley, RG: An Atlas of Surgical Approaches to the Bones of the Dog and Cat. WB Saunders Co., Philadelphia-London-Toronto 1966

Uhthoff, HK, Stahl, E: Current Concepts of Internal Fixation of Fractures. Springer-Verlag, Berlin-Heidelberg-New York 1980

Weber, BG, Brunner, C, Freuler, F: Treatment of Fractures in Children and Adolescents. Springer-Verlag, Berlin-Heidelberg-New York 1980

Subject Index

106

W. O. Brinker, R. B. Hohn, W. D. Prieur

Manual of Internal Fixation for Small Animals

1981. Approx. 550 figures. Approx. 350 pages
ISBN 3-540-10629-4
In preparation

Contents:
General Considerations: AO/ASIF Principles and techniques for fracture treatment, implants, pre- and postoperative care, infection and radiographic interpretation
Special Part: Internal fixation of fractures involving the various bones in the adult and immature animal.
Reconstructive Surgery: Delayed union and nonunion, osteotomy, arthrodesis and bone grafting.

All procedures covered in the Manual are supplemented by high quality illustrations, making it readily understandable. It has been written with the needs of the veterinary practitioner and student in mind.
The first part deals with AO/ASIF principles and methods of stable fixation. This includes function and main use of the different implants and instruments, operative technique, pre- and postoperative evaluation and care, metallurgy and postoperative complications. Also included is a discussion and treatment of delayed union, nonunion and reconstruction procedures (axial corrections, arthrodeses, bone grafting and transplantation).
A special section deals with proven methods of internal fixation for the most common fractures. It has been organized in anatomical sequence. These methods are all based on AO/ASIF principles of stable internal fixation and documentation records on numerous clinical cases.

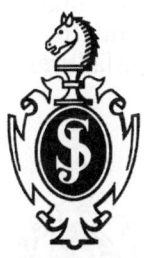
Springer-Verlag
Berlin
Heidelberg
New York

Manual of Internal Fixation

Techniques Recommended by the AO Group

By M. E. Müller, M. Allgöwer, R. Schneider, H. Willenegger
In collaboration with numerous experts
Translated from the German by J. Schatzker

2nd, expanded and revised edition. 1979.
345 figures in color, 2 Templates for Preoperative Planning. X, 409 pages
ISBN 3-540-09227-7

The second edition of this popular manual has been expanded and revised, facilitating full comprehension and flawless execution of internal fixation procedures. Particular attention is devoted in this edition to correlating the various fractures, their prognosis and the appropriate therapeutic technique.

The first section explains the basic biomechanic principles of the AO/ASIF method of stable internal fixation. It deals with the function and use of AO implants, AO instruments, and with the essentials of the operative technique and postoperative care. It also discusses the handling ot the most important postoperative complications.

The second section deals at length with the AO recommendations for operative treatment of the most common closed fractures in the adult. This is organized in anatomical sequence. A discussion of closed fractures is followed by a discussion of open fractures in the adult, then by one of fractures in children and finally, of pathological fractures.

The third part is a condensed presentation of the application of stable fixation to reconstructive bone surgery. An appendix is devoted to pseudarthroses, non-unions, and arthrodesès.

Based on clinical experience with over 50,000 operatively treated cases, this manual offers orthopedic surgeons, traumatologists, and general surgeons current and comprehensive information on this significantly successful technique.

AO/ASIF Instrumentation

F. Séquin, R. Texhammar

Manual of Use and Care

1981. Approx. 1300 figures, 17 separate instrument guides. Approx. 306 pages
ISBN 3-540-10337-6

The need for a partical guide to the use of AO instruments written with surgical assistants in mind has existed as long as the instruments themselves. This need is now met in AO/ASIF Instrumentation. It acquaints all members of the operating team with the goals and principles of AO/ASIF techniques while providing them with a comprehensive introduction to AO/ASIF instruments, their use and their maintenance. The book is arranged according to topic for easy reference, with carefully chosen illustrations rounding out the information in each section. Looseleaf tables are provided as checklists for laying out AO/ASIF instruments in the operating room.

AO/ASIF Instrumentation supplements two other volumes in the Springer-Verlag program – Manual of Internal Fixation and Small Fragment Set Manual – and contains

- explanations of the scientific and clinical significance of AO-ASIF techniques
- detailed descriptions of individual implants and instruments
- instructions for the handling and use of implants and instruments
- directions for the care and maintenance of AO/ASIF instruments.

This book will prove to be an indispensable reference for all surgical personnel concerned about the success of internal fixation and the avoidance of methodologically induced failures.

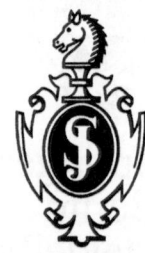

Springer-Verlag Berlin Heidelberg New York